Get Through
MRCP Part 2: 360 Best of Fives

To my mother and sister for all their support

Get Through

MRCP Part 2: 360 Best of Fives

Aruna Dias BSc MBBS MRCP (UK)
Specialist Registrar in Gastroenterology and
General Internal Medicine
Broomfield Hospital, Chelmsford, Essex

Editorial Adviser
Eric Beck FRCP (London, Glasgow and Edinburgh)

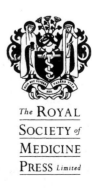

The ROYAL
SOCIETY of
MEDICINE
PRESS Limited

© 2004 Royal Society of Medicine Press Ltd

Published by the Royal Society of Medicine Press Ltd
1 Wimpole Street, London W1G 0AE, UK
Tel: +44 (0)20 7290 2921
Fax: +44 (0)20 7290 2929
E-mail: publishing@rsm.ac.uk
Website: www.rsmpress.co.uk

British Library Cataloguing in Publication Data
A catalogue record for this book is available from the British Library

ISBN 1-85315-527-6

Distribution in Europe and Rest of World:
Marston Book Services Ltd
PO Box 269
Abingdon
Oxon OX14 4YN, UK
Tel: +44 (0)1235 465500
Fax: +44 (0)1235 465555

Distribution in the USA and Canada:
Royal Society of Medicine Press Ltd
c/o Jamco Distribution Inc
1401 Lakeway Drive
Lewisville, TX 75057, USA
Tel: +1 800 538 1287
Fax: +1 972 353 1303
E-mail: jamco@majors.com

Distribution in Australia and New Zealand:
MacLennan + Petty Pty Ltd
Suite 405, 152 Bunnerong Road
Eastgardens NSW 2036
Australia
Tel: + 61 2 9349 5811
Fax: + 61 2 9349 5911

Phototypeset by Phoenix Photosetting, Chatham, Kent
Printed in Spain by T.G. Hostench S.A.

Contents

Acknowledgements

I am deeply indebted to the many SHOs, registrars and consultants at William Harvey Hospital, Ashford, Kent and Broomfield Hospital, Chelmsford, Essex for providing helpful suggestions and proof reading the text. In particular I would like to thank: Dawn Bayford, Graham Bradley, Ronan Breen, Selina Brewerton, Fateh Chowdhury, Stuart Coltart, Colley Crawford, Abhishek Deo, Jane Fisher, Jeremy Fletcher, Keith Hattatowa, Reena Joshi, Sam Khandhadia, Cho Cho Khin, Ilanga Samaratunga, John Sewell, Andrew Solomon, Arul Srinivasan, Robert Weir, Chula Wijesurendra, and Yiannis Zoukos.

The imaging questions in this book would not have been possible without the help given to me by the following:

Dr Peter Gishen of Hammersmith Hospital for allowing me to use his extensive collection of radiological imaging, Mrs Bunny Kallipetis of Kings College Hospital for helping to retrieve them and Dr Paras Dalal of St. Thomas' Hospital for reviewing all of the radiology questions with me.

Dr Mark Monaghan of Kings College Hospital for providing the echocardiograms.

Mrs Pamela Walsh and Mrs Sue Walker of the Paula Carr Trust, William Harvey Hospital, and the medical photography department of Broomfield Hospital for providing the ophthalmology pictures.

Dr Wendy Thurrell and Paul Williams of William Harvey Hospital for providing the histopathology imaging.

Dr James Nash of Public Health Laboratory Service, Ashford, Kent for providing the microbiology imaging.

Dr Catriona Irvine, of William Harvey Hospital and Dr Hilary Dodd, of Broomfield Hospital for providing the dermatology pictures.

Dr Koolan Nagendran of Broomfield Hospital for providing the neurophysiology pictures.

Dr Del Turner, of Broomfield Hospital and the coronary care units of Broomfield Hospital and William Harvey Hospital for providing the ECGs.

I would also like to thank Dr Una Coales, author of *Get Through MRCP Part 1*, for introducing me to the idea of doing this book; Dr Eric Beck, as a former examiner, for laboriously checking every single question and giving expert guidance on the format of the book; and Peter Altman and Peter Richardson of RSM Press for publishing this book and being very patient whilst I completed the task.

Recommended reading and references

Adair OV (2001) *Cardiology Secrets* 2nd edn. Philadelphia: Hanley & Belfus

Beck ER et al (2003) *Tutorials in Differential Diagnosis* 4th edn. Edinburgh: Churchill Livingstone

Bolognia JL et al (2003) *Dermatology* (2-volume set) London: Mosby

General Medical Council (2001) *Good Medical Practice* 3rd edn. London: GMC

Greenhalgh T (2001) *How to Read a Paper* 2nd edn. London: BMJ Publishing Group

Hoffbrand AV & Petit JE (2001) *Essential Haematology* 3rd edn. Oxford: Blackwell

Hricik DE et al (1999) *Nephrology Secrets*. Philadelphia: Hanley & Belfus

Kumar PJ & Clark M (2002) *Clinical Medicine*, 5th edn. London: Baillière Tindall

Ludlam CA (1990) *Clinical Haematology*. Edinburgh: Churchill Livingstone

McDermott MT (2001) *Endocrine Secrets* 3rd edn. Philadelphia: Hanley & Belfus

McNally PR (2001) *GI/Liver Secrets* 2nd edn. Philadelphia: Hanley & Belfus

Milner AD & Hull D (1998) *Hospital Paediatrics* 3rd edn. Edinburgh: Churchill Livingstone

Provan D et al (1998) *Oxford Handbook of Clinical Haematology*. Oxford: Oxford University Press

Ramrakha PS & Moore KP (1997) *Oxford Handbook of Acute Medicine*. Oxford: Oxford University Press

Rolak LA (2001) *Neurology Secrets* 3rd edn. Philadelphia: Hanley & Belfus

Royal Pharmaceutical Society of Great Britain (2003) *British National Formulary*. London: British Medical Association

Ryder REJ et al (1999) *An Aid to the MRCP Short Cases* 2nd edn. Oxford: Blackwell

Schiller KFR et al (2001) *Atlas of Gastrointestinal Endoscopy and Related Pathology*. Oxford: Blackwell

West SG (2002) *Rheumatology Secrets* 2nd edn. Philadelphia: Hanley & Belfus

Wood ME (1999) *Haematology/Oncology Secrets* 2nd edn. Philadelphia: Hanley & Belfus

Reference values

HAEMATOLOGY

Haemoglobin (HB)	Male	13.0–18.0 g/dL
	Female	11.5–16.5 g/dL
MCH		28–32 pg
MCV		80–96 fL
MCHC		32–35 g/dL
White cell count (WCC)	Total	$4–11 \times 10^9$/L
	Neutrophils	$1.5–7 \times 10^9$/L
	Lymphocytes	$1.5–4 \times 10^9$/L
	Monocytes	$0–0.8 \times 10^9$/L
	Eosinophils	$0.04–0.4 \times 10^9$/L
	Basophils	$0–0.1 \times 10^9$/L
Platelets		$150–400 \times 10^9$/L
Reticulocyte count		0.5–2.5%
ESR	Male	0–20 mm/1st hr
	Female	0–30 mm/1st hr

CLOTTING

Activated partial thromboplastin time/APTT	30–40 s
Bleeding time	3–8 minutes
D-Dimer	<1 mg/L
Factor II, V, VII, VIII, IX, X, XI, XII	50–150 IU/dL
Fibrinogen degradation products/FDP	<100 mg/L
Fibrinogen	1.8–5.4 g/L
INR	<1.4
Prothrombin time/PT	11.5–15.5 s
Von Willebrand factor	45–150 IU/dL

BIOCHEMISTRY

Alanine aminotransferase (ALT)	5–35 U/L
Albumin	37–49 g/L
Aldosterone	
Supine	135–400 pmol/L
Upright	330–830 pmol/L
Alkaline phosphatase (ALP)	45–105 U/L (over 14 years age)
Ammonia (Plasma)	12–55 mol/L
Amylase	60–180 U/L
Anion gap	12–16 mmol/L
Aspartate aminotransferase (AST)	1–31 U/L
Bicarbonate	22–30 mmol/L
Bilirubin	
Total	1–22 mmol/L
Conjugated	0–3.4 mmol/L
C-reactive protein	<10 mg/L
Caeruloplasmin	200–350 mg/L

Calcitonin	<27 pmol/L
Calcium (corrected)	2.2–2.6 mmol/L
Chloride	95–107 mmol/L
Cholesterol	
Total	<5.2 mmol/L
LDL Cholesterol	<3.36 mmol/L
HDL Cholesterol	>1.55 mmol/L
Cholecalciferol/25-Vitamin D_3	60–105 nmol/L
25-OH-Cholecalciferol/ 1,25-Vitamin D_3	45–90 nmol/L
Complement	
C_3	65–190 mg/dL
C_4	15–50 mg/dL
Copper	12–26 mol/L
Creatine kinase	
Males	25–195 U/L
Females	35–170 U/L
Creatinine	60–110 mmol/L
Ferritin	15–300 g/L
Folate	
Serum	2.0–11.0 g/L
Red cell	160–640 g/L
Gamma glutamyl transferase (GGT)	4–35 U/L
Gastrin	<55 pmol/L
Globulin	23–35 g/L
Glucose (plasma)	
Fasting normal	3.0–6.0 mmol/L
Haemoglobin A_1C	3.8–6.4 %
Haptoglobin	0.13–1.63 g/L
Immunoglobulins	
IgA	0.8–3.0 g/L
IgG	6.0–13.0 g/L
IgM	0.4–2.5 g/L
IgE	<120 kU/L
Iron	12–30 mol/L
Lactate (Plasma)	0.6–1.8 mmol/L
Lactate dehydrogenase (LDH)	10–250 U/L
Magnesium	0.75–1.05 mmol/L
Osmolality (Plasma)	278–305 mosmol/Kg
Parathyroid hormone/PTH (Plasma)	0.9–5.4 pmol/L
Phosphate	0.8–1.4 mmol/L
Potassium (K)	3.5–5.0 mmol/L
Prolactin (Plasma)	<360 mU/L
Protein	60–76 g/L
PTH-related peptide	<1.8 pmol/L
Renin (Plasma)	
Supine	1.1–2.7 pmol/ml/hour
Upright	3.0–4.3 pmol/ml/hour
Sodium (Na)	135–145 mmol/L
Thyroid binding globulin (Plasma)	13–28 mg/L
Thyroid stimulating hormone/TSH (Plasma)	0.4–5 mU/L

Thyroxine (Plasma)
Total T_4 58–174 nmol/L
    Free T_4 10–25 pmol/L
    Total T_3 1.07–3.18 nmol/L
    Free T_3 5–10 pmol/L
Total iron binding capacity (TIBC)   45–75 mol/L
Transferrin   2.0–4.0 g/L
Triglyceride   0.45–1.69 mmol/L
Troponin I   <0.4 g/L
Troponin T   <0.1 g/L
Urate
    Males   0.23–0.46 mmol/L
    Females   0.19–0.36 mmol/L
Urea   2.5–7.5 mmol/L
Vitamin B_{12} 160–760 ng/L

BLOOD GASES
H^+ 35–45 nmol/L
pH   7.35–7.45
P_aCO_2 4.7–6.0 kPa
P_aO_2 11.3–12.6 kPa
Base Excess   ± 2 mmol/L
Carboxyhaemoglobin
    Non-smoker   <2 %
    Smoker   3–15 %

CSF
Cell count
    Neutrophils   None
    Lymphocytes   60–70 %
    Monocytes   30–50 %
Protein   0.15–0.45 g/L
Glucose   3.3–4.4 mmol/L
Opening pressure   5–18 cm H_2O

URINE
5-Hydroxyindolacetic acid (5-HIAA)   10–47 mol/24 hours
Adrenaline   <144 nmol/24 hours
Albumin   <30 mg/24 hours
Calcium   2.5–7.5 mmol/24 hours
Dopamine   <3100 nmol/24 hours
Glomerular filtration rate   70–140 ml/min
Noradrenaline   <570 nmol/24 hours
Osmolality   350–1000 mosmol/Kg
Protein   <0.2 g/24 hours
Vanillyl mandelic acid (VMA)   5–35 mol/24 hours

List of abbreviations

ACE	angiotensin-converting enzyme
ACTH	adrenocorticotrophic hormone
ADH	antidiuretic hormone
ARDS	adult respiratory distress syndrome
ALP	alkaline phosphatase
ALT	alanine aminotransferase
ANA	antinuclear antibody
ANCA	antineutrophil cytoplasm antibody
APS	autoimmune polyglandular syndrome
APTT	activated partial thromboplastin time
ARR	absolute risk reduction
AST	aspartate transaminase
AV	atrioventricular
AZT	azidothymidine
C	complement
CA	cancer antigen
CD	cluster designation
CJD	Creutzfeldt–Jakob disease
CK	creatine kinase
COPD	chronic obstructive pulmonary disease
CSF	cerebrospinal fluid
CT	computed tomography
CRP	C-reactive protein
CVP	central venous pressure
DDAVP	1-deamino-8-D-vasopressin
DEXA	dual-energy X ray absorptiometry
DKA	diabetic ketoacidosis
DLCO	carbon monoxide diffusion in the lung
DS-DNA	double-stranded deoxyribonucleic acid
ECG	electrocardiogram, -graphy
EEG	electroencephalogram, -graphy
ERCP	endoscopic retrograde cholangiopancreatography
ESR	erythrocyte sedimentation rate
FEV_1	forced expiratory volume in 1 second
FiO_2	fractional concentration of oxygen in inspired gas
FOB	faecal occult blood
FSGS	focal segmental glomerulosclerosis
FSH	follicle-stimulating hormone
FVC	forced vital capacity
G6PD	glucose-6-phosphate dehydrogenase
GBM	glomerular basement membrane
GCS	Glasgow coma scale
GGT	γ-glutamyltransferase
GI	gastrointestinal
HAART	highly active antiretroviral treatment
Hb	haemoglobin
HBcAg	hepatitis B core antigen

HBeAg	hepatitis B e antigen
HBsAg	hepatitis B surface antigen
HCG	human chorionic gonadotrophin
HCV	hepatitis C virus
HDL	high density lipoprotein
5-HIAA	5-hydroxyindoleacetic acid
HIV	human immunodeficiency virus
HOCM	hypertrophic obstructive cardiomyopathy
HSMN	hereditary motor and sensory neuropathy
HSP	Henoch–Schönlein purpura
Ig	immunoglobulin
IDDM	insulin dependent diabetes mellitus
INR	international normalised ratio
ITP	idiopathic thrombocytopenic purpura
JVP	jugular venous pressure
K	potassium
KCO	diffusion coefficient
LBBB	left bundle branch block
LDH	lactate dehydrogenase
LDL	low density lipoprotein
LH	luteinising hormone
MCV	mean corpuscular volume
MEN	multiple endocrine neoplasia
MI	myocardial infarction
MRCP	magnetic resonance cholangiopancreatography
MRI	magnetic resonance imaging
Na	sodium
NNT	number needed to treat
OR	odds ratio
PAWP	pulmonary artery wedge pressure
PCO_2	partial pressure of carbon dioxide
PCR	polymerase chain reaction
PCV	polycythaemia rubra vera
PO_2	partial pressure of oxygen
PEG	percutaneous endoscopic gastrostomy
PRV	polycythaemia rubra vera
PT	prothrombin time
PTC	percutaneous transhepatic cholangiogram, -graphy
PTH	parathyroid hormone
RBBB	right bundle branch block
RCT	randomised control trial
RNA	ribonucleic acid
RTA	renal tubular acidosis
SIADH	syndrome of inappropriate ADH secretion
SLE	systemic lupus erythematosus
T_3	tri-iodothyronine
T_4	thyroxine
TB	tuberculosis
TLC	total lung capacity
TPA	tissue plasminogen activator
TSH	thyroid-stimulating hormone

TT	thrombin time
VIP	vasointestinal peptide
VMA	vanillylmandelic acid
VT/VF	ventricular tachycardia/ventricular fibrillation
WCC	white cell count
WPW	Wolff–Parkinson–White

Introduction

The MRCP (UK) examination is now an obstacle that, in the UK, has to be passed after a statutory minimum period of prescribed general medical training, before a candidate can pursue higher specialist training. Finding the time to study whilst dealing with on-call duties, shift patterns, ward work, not forgetting other aspects of social life, is not an easy task.

The examination has changed radically leaving the many guides and manuals designed for the previous MRCP (UK) out of date. Although no book can guarantee you will have every answer at your fingertips, it can help you to make best use of your knowledge by familiarising you with new formats illustrated by copious examples. Hence the newly devised series by the RSM Press: 'Get Through MRCP'.

As you will know, having passed Part 1, the previous multiple True/False MCQs in it have been replaced by single best answer MCQs. Generally, a stem will have five completions each having some degree of correctness/plausibility and the task is to choose the SINGLE best answer (hence best of five/BOF). Rarely the completions may be extended to ten or fifteen and two or three answers have to be chosen. A correct answer earns 1 mark; there is no longer negative marking for a wrong answer in the Part 1 paper (there never was in Part 2). Hence a candidate is no longer penalised for guessing – make what you wish of that! Furthermore the pass rate is no longer predetermined as a fixed percentage of candidates (peer reference). Rather a predetermined standard is set by the examiners and all candidates achieving it will pass (criterion reference). Candidates are no longer directly competing with each other.

The details of criterion referencing/standard setting in Parts 1 and 2 have not yet been made public. In this book (as in the companion volume for Part 1 by Una Coales) the degree of perceived difficulty of each question is graded on a three point scale, making a judgement on what proportion of candidates just passing the whole examination are likely to get that particular question right, viz:

*	20–50% 'just passing' candidates expected to get correct
**	50–75% 'just passing' candidates expected to get correct
***	75–100% 'just passing' candidates expected to get correct

Thus an easier paper will require a higher mark to pass as shown in the accompanying table where the notional pass marks in the six papers in the book range from 56–63%. (Note that 'blind guessing' gives up to a 1 in 5 or 20% chance of being correct!).

Criterion referencing of 6 papers in the book (note that although there are 60 questions in each a few questions are extended, requiring two or three answers).

Paper	Difficulty of Questions			Passmark	% mark
	*	**	***		
1	13	36	13	39/62	63
2	17	33	14	39/64	61
3	13	38	10	38/61	62
4	9	37	14	38/60	63
5	15	39	6	35/60	58
6	21	34	6	34/61	56

Since the content of the final Part 2 examination – PACES (Practical Assessment of Clinical Examination Skills) differs from the previous traditional Long Case – Short Case – Oral format, certain topics are no longer examined there, but appear in the extended written papers instead. Thus the all important medical emergencies, evidence based medicine, long term management of chronic disease, critical reading, application of statistical methods, psychological aspects of illness, to name some, will now appear in Part 1 and, particularly, in Part 2 written papers instead. This is clearly reflected in the book. Furthermore the new Part 2 papers are no longer artificially subdivided into case history, data interpretation and photographic material. Again this is reflected in over one third of the questions in each paper being illustrated by colour photographs, ECGs and echocardiograms or other forms of imaging.

As the questions are now multiple choice a much wider syllabus is covered and questions can be asked from different angles. Examiners setting questions go to great lengths to avoid ambiguity in their wording. However, sometimes an answer may be so blindingly obvious that it would be difficult to find four plausible distracters; look out for the occasional format of: 'Every answer is true except for . . .'. It is rare for there to be more than one part to a question as there would often be linkage between questions asking for 'best diagnosis', 'best investigation' and 'best treatment'. Rather, the question may appear in a different examination with a different completion. Although it was sometimes considered in the past that esoteric knowledge was being (unfairly) tested in the 'open page' format, where candidates had to dredge the knowledge from an already overloaded memory, now if rarities are asked, candidates will be prompted by seeing them as an option in front of them; judgment is being tested in Part 2 of knowledge already acquired in passing Part 1.

Generally, in answering the questions, think of what answer you would give before looking at each distracter. If you find your answer amongst them you are probably right and need not waste valuable time weighing up the pros and cons of each distracter in turn. Incidentally, the order in which they appear is usually alphabetical so do not look for patterns of favoured responses in the ABCDE – they do not exist. Sometimes however, particularly, with management options you may have, as in real life, to weigh up what is best for the patient in the question.

In the interests of uncluttered reading you will find at the beginning a list of abbreviations used throughout the book and in everyday life. You will also find a list of normal values with only a few given in the text. Increasingly there is a standardisation of test methods but enzymes and hormone measurement reference values may still vary.

Finally, the answers section gives you detailed explanations not only why one is the best but also why the others are less good. We hope you will find this a useful and pleasurable form of programmed learning even if you do not always agree with everything written. The index will help to locate particular points.

We hope you enjoy the book as much as we did when compiling it – and good luck in the exam.

Paper I

Questions

1.1 A 60-year-old man with a history of congestive cardiac failure and mild asthma presented with worsening shortness of breath that was now occurring at rest. He could walk only 20 metres on flat ground and could only manage six stairs before having to stop to catch his breath. He had no chest pain. He slept with three pillows at night. He stopped smoking over 30 years ago and did not drink alcohol.

On examination his pulse was 72 regular and his blood pressure was 155/90. Jugular venous pressure was elevated to 4 cm above the sternal angle. Heart sounds were normal and there were no murmurs. His chest was clear and his respiratory rate was 18 breaths/min.

Oxygen saturation on air was 94% and peak flow was 300 L/min.

He was currently on furosemide (frusemide) 80 mg o.d., enalapril 20 mg o.d. and salbutamol inhaler.

Bloods	Hb	15.0	WCC	10.0
	Platelets	300	Na	130
	K	4.2	Urea	5.8
	Creatinine	100		

Echocardiogram	Mild tricuspid regurgitation
	No evidence of pulmonary hypertension
	Severe left ventricular systolic dysfunction
	Ejection fraction 35%

The most appropriate management for this patient would be to:

A add in digoxin
B add in low dose atenolol
C add in low dose spironolactone
D change furosemide (frusemide) to co-amilofruse
E increase furosemide (frusemide) to b.d.

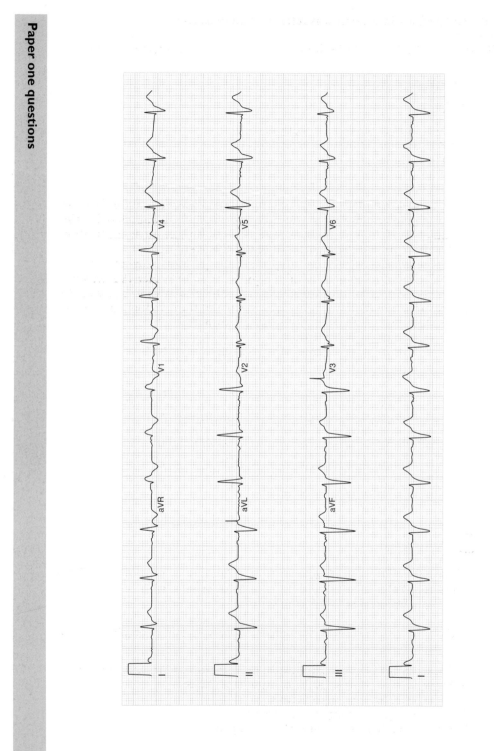

1.2 An 84-year-old woman was referred with dizziness.

PR interval 0.28 s; QRS duration 0.16 s; QT interval 0.28 s.

Her ECG shows:

    A LBBB
    B RBBB
    C RBBB and left anterior fascicular block
    D RBBB and left posterior fascicular block
    E trifascicular block + P-Rhut p

1.3 A 19-year-old woman was admitted with a salicylate overdose. She had taken 40 tablets 16 hours ago. She complained of abdominal pain, vomiting, tinnitus and sweating. She was not on any other medication and had not drunk alcohol at the time of the overdose.

On examination she was hyperventilating. Her temperature was 38.0°C, pulse 98 regular and blood pressure 100/60. Her JVP was not elevated and heart sounds were normal. Her respiratory rate was 30 breaths/min and her chest was clear. She had diffuse abdominal tenderness. There was no focal neurological abnormality.

Bloods	Hb	13.8	WCC	10.0
	Platelets	180	INR	1.1
	Na	135	K	5.8
	Urea	19.8	Creatinine	240
	Protein	70	Albumin	39
	Bilirubin	14	ALT	55
	ALP	90	GGT	39
	Glucose	3.0		

Paracetamol	Not detected			
Salicylate	530 mg/L			

Arterial blood gases on air	pH	7.21	PCO_2	2.1
	PO_2	10.4	Bicarbonate	10.2
	Base excess	−15.4		

Which **ONE** of the following statements concerning her management is correct?

    A Development of convulsions would be an indication for haemodialysis
    B Forced alkaline diuresis is the treatment of choice
    C Pyrexia suggests underlying sepsis
    D Immediate gastric lavage should be given
    E Intravenous N-acetylcysteine should be given

1.4 A 4-year-old boy presented with sudden onset fever and painful oral lesions (Figure 1.4). See plate section.

The most likely organism to have caused this is:

A *Candida albicans*
B *Herpes simplex virus*
C *Molluscum contagiosum*
D *Staphylococcus aureus*
E *Streptococcus pyogenes*

1.5 A 55-year-old woman complained of pain in her legs and difficulty in walking over the past 2 months. She had a previous medical history of insulin dependent diabetes and had recently been diagnosed as having coeliac disease.

On examination her pulse was 72 regular and blood pressure 154/90. Her chest was clear and abdominal examination was normal. She had no rash. Her lower limb muscles were tender and there was weakness of her quadriceps and hip girdle muscles but no wasting. There was normal tone, power, reflexes and sensation.

Bloods	Hb	12.2	MCV	101.3
	WCC	6.7	Platelets	325
	Na	144	K	4.5
	Urea	3.7	Creatinine	100
	Calcium	1.99	Phosphate	0.6
	ALP	140	Albumin	38
	Protein	70	Glucose	10.5
	HbA$_{1c}$	7.5%		

The most likely cause of her symptoms is:

A diabetic amyotrophy
B osteomalacia
C osteoporosis
D periodic paralysis
E peripheral neuropathy

1.6 It has been proposed that continued excessive alcohol intake is associated with the development of stomach carcinoma. You have been asked to design a study to investigate this possibility.

The most appropriate study design would be:

A case control study
B case reports
C cohort study
D cross-sectional study
E randomised control trial

1.7 A 55-year-old Caucasian woman with Crohn's disease presented with back pain. She had not had any falls. She had had numerous courses of prednisolone in the past but was not on hormone replacement therapy. A DEXA scan was performed and she has returned wanting to know the result.

DEXA scan of total hip   T score   −1.5
                                Z score   −1.6

The interpretation of the DEXA scan result is:

A normal bone mass
B osteopenia appropriate for her age
C osteopenia inappropriate for her age
D osteoporosis appropriate for her age
E osteoporosis inappropriate for her age

1.8 A 13-year-old boy presented to Accident & Emergency with severe generalised bruising following a fall. Apart from a sore throat 1 week ago, he had no previous medical history.

On examination he was apyrexial. Physical examination was normal apart from bruising all over his body and limbs. There was no lymphadenopathy.

Bloods	Hb	12.9	MCV	78
	WCC	11.3	Platelets	15
	Neutrophils	5.8	Lymphocytes	5.1
	Monocytes	0.4		

The most likely diagnosis is:

A acute lymphoblastic leukaemia
B acute myeloid leukaemia
C aplastic anaemia
D idiopathic thrombocytopenic purpura
E Henoch–Schönlein purpura

1.9 A 16-year-old girl presented to Accident & Emergency with abdominal pain. She had had recurrent attacks in the past. The pain was generalised and was associated with nausea and shortness of breath. Until now the pain had resolved spontaneously but could last for hours. She had no bowel or urinary problems. She was not pregnant. Her mother used to suffer similar problems as a teenager.

On examination she was in pain. Her temperature was 37.0°C, pulse 120 regular and blood pressure 130/70. Her respiratory rate was 24 breaths per minute and chest was clear. There was generalised abdominal tenderness but bowel sounds were present. Rectal examination was normal.

Bloods	Hb	13.5	WCC	7.8
	Platelets	190	Na	140
	K	4.4	Urea	4.8
	Creatinine	80	Protein	74
	Albumin	42	Bilirubin	12
	ALT	25	ALP	85
	Amylase	50	Ca	2.25
	Phosphate	0.9	ESR	12
	CRP	10		

Urinanalysis No protein, glucose or white cells. HCG negative

Chest X-ray Normal

CT abdomen Some localised oedema in proximal jejunum

Laparoscopy No abnormalities detected

The most likely diagnosis is:

A acute intermittent porphyria
B familial Mediterranean fever
C hereditary angioedema
D polyarteritis nodosa
E Wiskott–Aldrich syndrome

1.10 A 72-year-old man presented with a 4-day history of severe abdominal pain and diarrhoea with some blood mixed with stool. He opened his bowels up to 7-8 times per day. He had a normal appetite but had lost some weight. Five days ago he had been discharged from hospital with an infective exacerbation of chronic obstructive pulmonary disease, where his treatment included steroids, nebulisers and antibiotics. He had no recent foreign travel.

On examination his temperature was 37.5°C, pulse 92 regular and blood pressure 123/88. Chest was clear. His abdomen was generally tender but there was no organomegaly. Flexible sigmoidoscopy was performed and biopsies were taken (Figure 1.10). See plate section.

The most likely diagnosis is:

A colorectal carcinoma
B Crohn's disease
C acute diverticulitis
D ischaemic colitis
E pseudomembranous colitis

1.11 A 28-year-old man presented with a 7-day history of fever, watery diarrhoea and abdominal pain and now had also developed a dry cough. He had returned from South Africa 5 days ago where he had been on safari. He had no previous medical problems, was on no medication, and did not take malaria prophylaxis.

On examination he had a few cervical lymph nodes. His temperature was 39.0°C, pulse 64 regular and blood pressure 118/76. JVP was not elevated and heart sounds and chest were normal. His abdomen was soft and he had 2 cm non-tender hepatomegaly.

Bloods				
	Hb	12.9	WCC	2.4
	Neutrophils	1.3	Lymphocytes	1.0
	Eosinophils	0.1	Platelets	219
	Na	139	K	4.2
	Urea	3.8	Creatinine	78
	Protein	65	Albumin	35
	Bilirubin	13	ALT	25
	ALP	100	ESR	36
	CRP	43	INR	1.1

Malaria films Negative

Urinanalysis Normal

Chest X-ray Normal

The most likely diagnosis is:

A amoebic dysentery
B blackwater fever
C dengue haemorrhagic fever
D typhoid
E yellow fever

1.12 A 24-year-old woman presented with a 6-week history of headache and blurred vision and this had affected her job. There was no significant previous medical history. She did not smoke and drank half a bottle of wine at the weekend. The headache begins at the back of her head and was associated with flashing lights and zigzag lines. There was no vomiting, falls or fits. Her appetite and weight were stable. There was no family history of migraine. Apart from the combined oral contraceptive pill she was on no medication.

She was apyrexial, pulse 90 regular and blood pressure 142/84. Respiratory and neck examinations were normal. Examination of her cranial nerves and her peripheral nervous system was unremarkable. Fundoscopic examination was performed (Figure 1.12). See plate section.

Bloods	Hb	13.8	WCC	5.8
	Platelets	190	ESR	8
	Na	141	K	4.6
	Urea	4.7	Creatinine	46
	CRP	13	PT	11.9
	APTT	30		

CT brain   Normal

The most helpful investigation would be:

A cerebral angiography
B EEG
C lumbar puncture
D magnetic resonance venography
E thrombophilia screen

1.13 A 35-year-old woman with IDDM was referred with recent onset blurred vision. Fundoscopy was performed (Figure 1.13). See plate section.

The most likely cause of her worsening vision is:

A branch retinal artery occlusion
B branch retinal vein occlusion
C diabetic maculopathy
D traction retinal detachment
E vitreous haemorrhage

1.14 A 65-year-old man had a colonoscopy to investigate the cause of his rectal bleeding. At the rectosigmoid junction a large ulcerated mass was found that extended halfway into the diameter of the lumen and bled readily on contact. A barium enema showed no other mass in his large intestine and abdominal ultrasound revealed no liver metastases. He had a sigmoid colectomy. Histology of the mass revealed poorly differentiated adenocarcinoma with invasion through the serosa but no regional lymph node involvement.

Using the modified Dukes' classification system, this patient's tumour would be graded as:

A Dukes' A
B Dukes' B$_1$
C Dukes' B$_2$
D Dukes' C$_1$
E Dukes' C$_2$

1.15 A 44-year-old man presented with a 2-day history of painful, swollen left knee. It came on gradually and there was no history of trauma. He did not have a history of joint pain or any other previous medical history. He was not on any medication. On examination he was in pain. His temperature was 37.0°C, pulse 98 regular and blood pressure 130/88. Cardiovascular and respiratory examinations were normal. His left knee was swollen, erythematous and tender with an obvious effusion but normal range of movements. There was no rash and tone, power, reflexes and sensation were normal.

Bloods	Hb	13.6	WCC	9.2
	Neutrophils	6.5	Platelets	348
	Na	138	K	4.3
	Urea	3.5	Creatinine	68
	ESR	24	CRP	49

Blood cultures No growth

Rheumatoid factor Negative

Left knee X-ray Soft tissue swelling
No fracture

Synovial fluid Slightly turbid appearance
WCC   35,000   Neutrophils 60%
Protein   35
Crystals showing negative birefringence

The most likely diagnosis is:

A bacterial septic arthritis
B gout
C osteoarthritis
D palindromic rheumatoid arthritis
E pseudogout

1.16 A 19-year-old student was admitted with headache, photophobia and malaise for one-day. She had no previous medical history and was not on any medication. On examination she was drowsy with a temperature of 38.5°C, pulse 110 regular and blood pressure 90/55. JVP was not elevated and heart sounds were normal. Cranial nerve examination was normal and there was no focal neurological deficit. There was a non-blanching rash on her legs (Figure 1.16). See plate section.

The **LEAST** appropriate step in the immediate management of this patient would be:

    A inform consultant in charge of communicable diseases for tracing of close contacts
    B intravenous aciclovir
    C intravenous cefotaxime
    D lumbar puncture if clotting and platelet count are normal
    E nasal and throat swabs for microbiological analysis

1.17 A 55-year-old man presented with collapse. His GCS at the time of presentation was 14/15 (Figure 1.17). See plate section.

The CT scan shows:

    A left cerebral abscess
    B left extradural haematoma
    C left intracerebral haemorrhage
    D left subdural haematoma
    E subarachnoid haemorrhage

1.18 A 52-year-old woman presented with a 3-month history of progressive dysphagia and weight loss. (Fig 1.18)

The most likely diagnosis is:

    A achalasia
    B benign stricture
    C carcinoma of the oesophagus
    D oesophageal candidiasis
    E oesophageal varices

1.19 A 51-year-old woman was admitted with an anterior MI. She was treated with TPA. She made an uneventful recovery.

Which **THREE** of the following medications/classes of medication have **NOT** been shown conclusively to improve prognosis post-MI?

    A ACE inhibitors
    B Aspirin
    C Atenolol
    D Calcium antagonists
    E Clopidogrel
    F Low molecular weight heparin
    G N3 polyunsaturated fat fish oils
    H Nicorandil
    I Nitrates
    J Simvastatin

1.20 A 75-year-old man was referred for a pacemaker check because he complained of dizziness. He had no chest pain or shortness of breath. He had a previous history of myocardial infarction 10 years ago. He had a permanent pacemaker fitted 2 years ago for complete heart block. He was only on aspirin. His pulse was 60 paced and blood pressure 116/58. His JVP was not elevated and both heart sounds were normal.

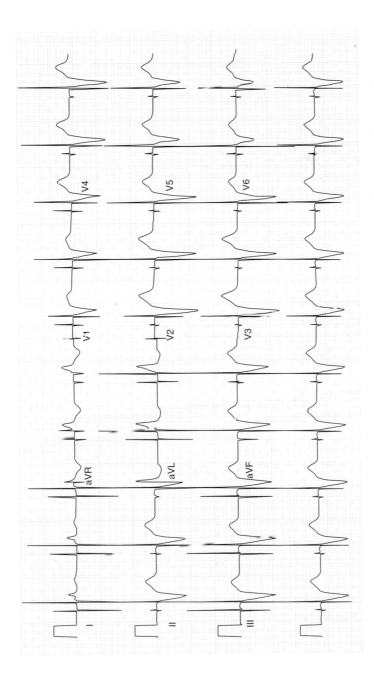

Which **ONE** of the following statements concerning this patient is true?

    A Anaemia can alter the rate of the pacemaker
    B He is likely to have a VVI pacemaker
    C His pacemaker is malfunctioning and that is the cause of his dizziness
    D Pyrexia can alter the rate of the pacemaker
    E When he had his original pacemaker fitted he was likely to have been in atrial fibrillation

1.21 A 25-year-old man was brought in to the Accident & Emergency department after attempting suicide by inhalation of carbon monoxide. He had a headache and had vomited three times. He had no past medical problems and was not on any medication. He did not drink alcohol or smoke.

On examination he was drowsy and there was a red discoloration around his cheeks and some blueness of his lips. His pulse was 110 regular and blood pressure 100/74. His JVP was not elevated and heart sounds were normal. His respiratory rate was 24 breaths/min and his chest was clear. Abdominal examination was normal. There were no focal neurological abnormalities.

Arterial blood gases on air	pH	7.40	PCO_2	2.9
	PO_2	12.4	Bicarbonate	24

Base excess 1.0

Carbon monoxide 30%

Which **ONE** of the following statements concerning this patient's condition is true?

    A A high PCO_2 is associated with a worse prognosis
    B Carbon monoxide causes the oxygen-dissociation curve to shift to the right
    C Development of focal neurological signs would be an indication for hyperbaric oxygen therapy
    D Intravenous doxapram would improve his condition
    E Pulse oximetery is an accurate measure of carboxyhaemoglobin (COHb)

1.22 A 29-year-old woman presented with a non-pruritic skin rash on her back, shoulders and arms. Ten days ago she had a bout of tonsillitis (Figure 1.22). See plate section.

The most likely diagnosis is:

    A guttate psoriasis
    B lichen planus
    C pityriasis versicolor
    D tinea corporis
    E pityriasis rosea

1.23 A 30-year-old woman who was 15 weeks pregnant developed sweating and tachycardia. She also complained about diplopia and a swelling in her neck.

    On examination she had a temperature of 37.3°C, pulse 110 regular and blood pressure 140/65. She had a tender, smooth enlarged goitre and exophthalmus.

Bloods	TSH	<0.1	Free T$_4$	45
	Free T$_3$	18		

The most appropriate treatment for this patient would be:

A atenolol
B prednisolone
C propylthiouracil
D iodine-131
E thyroidectomy

1.24 Two thousand patients with stroke were randomly allocated to treatment with either aspirin or placebo. At the end of 1 year five patients in the aspirin group had died, compared with 15 of the placebo group.

The number needed to treat (NNT) to prevent one death is:

A 5
B 15
C 75
D 100
E 200

1.25 A 75-year-old woman was referred with black stools. It was late at night when she presented to Accident & Emergency. She had recently been started on diclofenac for osteoarthritis. There was no haematemesis but she had passed approximately 400 ml of dark motions today. She had no other medical problems and was not taking any other medication. She did not drink alcohol.

    On examination she was apyrexial. Her pulse was 98 regular and blood pressure 120/70 with no postural drop. Abdominal examination revealed some epigastric tenderness but no guarding and bowel sounds were present. Rectal examination revealed fresh melaena.

Bloods	Hb	11.4	WCC	9.6
	Platelets	500	INR	1.2
	Na	139	K	4.5
	Urea	7.8	Creatinine	85
	Albumin	40	Protein	70
	Bilirubin	19	AST	26
	ALP	100	Amylase	95

Chest X-ray No free gas under the diaphragm

Abdominal X-ray No evidence of obstruction

Of the following, the next step in the immediate management would be:

    A immediate upper gastrointestinal endoscopy
    B intravenous omeprazole
    C intravenous propranolol
    D intravenous ranitidine
    E intravenous terlipressin

1.26 A 42-year-old woman was admitted with ascites, which had been increasing over the past 2 months. She also complained of progressive lethargy and that her skin bruised easily. Her urine was dark but stools were normal coloured. She did not drink alcohol, had no previous medical history and was on no medication.

    On examination she looked pale. She was apyrexial and there was no lymphadenopathy. Her pulse was 94 regular and blood pressure 110/75. Her abdomen was distended with generalised tenderness and there was 3 cm hepatomegaly.

Bloods	Hb	8.9	MCV	76.4
	WCC	2.9	Platelets	98
	Na	140	K	4.3
	Urea	5.9	Creatinine	90
	Protein	65	Albumin	32
	Bilirubin	18	ALT	65
	ALP	100	INR	1.1

Abdominal ultrasound Hepatomegaly with enlarged caudate lobe

                       No flow in hepatic veins

                       Gross ascites

The most helpful test to establish the underlying diagnosis would be:

A bone marrow aspirate and trephine
B haemoglobin electrophoresis
C Ham's test
D osmotic fragility studies
E Schumm's test

1.27 A 55-year-old man was referred with hepatomegaly and deranged liver function tests. He did not drink alcohol and had no risk factors for hepatitis. He had a previous medical history of rheumatoid arthritis, which affected his hands, elbows and knees. He was on no medication. He had a normal appetite and stable weight.

On examination he was not jaundiced or pale. His pulse was 79 regular and blood pressure 140/89. Respiratory examination was normal. He had 6 cm hepatomegaly but no other signs of chronic liver disease.

Bloods				
	Hb	13.4	WCC	4.5
	Platelets	110	INR	1.4
	Na	132	K	4.8
	Urea	3.9	Creatinine	80
	Albumin	33	Protein	70
	Bilirubin	30	ALT	85
	ALP	105	GGT	39
	Glucose	5.4		

Hepatitis A, B,
C serology   Negative

Liver biopsy (H&E) (Figure 1.27). See plate section.

The most likely diagnosis is:

A α_1-antitrypsin deficiency
B amyloidosis
C haemochromatosis
D hepatocellular carcinoma
E Wilson's disease

1.28 A 45-year-old man known to have contracted HIV was referred for HAART. In the past year he had developed lobar pneumonia due to *Steptococcus pneumoniae*. He had no other medical problems but continued to inject heroin. He was hepatitis B and C negative. He had a normal appetite and his weight was stable. Apart from oral candidiasis, no abnormalities were found on physical examination.

Bloods   Hb   11.4   WCC   3.9

Platelets   150

CD4   450

Viral load 16,000

Which **ONE** of the following statements concerning his management is correct?

A Zidovudine (AZT) should be avoided in anaemic patients
B He should be treated with long-term septrin
C Oral candidiasis would be an indication to start HAART
D Standard HAART treatment consists of two drugs
E Viral load is the most important determinant of when to start HAART

1.29 A 47-year-old gentleman presented with inability to walk. His problem started yesterday with weakness but now he could not stand. He had not opened his bowels yet. He was able to use his arms normally and there were no problems with his eyes or swallowing but he had some shortness of breath on exertion. Two weeks ago he had had salmonella gastro-enteritis. There was no previous medical history and he was not on any medication.

On examination he was anxious. His pulse was 120 regular and blood pressure 130/94. Respiratory examination was normal. There was no palpable bladder; normal anal tone. There was no muscle wasting or fasciculation. In the lower limbs tone was decreased, power was 0/5 and reflexes were absent. There was decreased sensation in the distal lower limbs. Upper limbs and cranial nerve examination were normal.

Bloods   Hb   12.8   WCC   7.4

Platelets   223   ESR   36

Glucose   5.6

CSF   Glucose   3.6   Protein   1.7 g/L

WCC   5

Poor prognosis would be associated with the presence or development of:

A *Escherichia coli* infection
B loss of reflexes and sensory involvement
C low peak expiratory flow rate
D low vital capacity
E *Salmonella typhi* infection

1.30 A 45-year-old woman was admitted with decreased level of consciousness. No history was available.

Arterial blood gases on air	pH	7.25	PCO_2	3.5
	PO_2	7.9		
	Bicarbonate	15.6	Base excess	−7.6

These blood gases show:

    A metabolic acidosis and type I respiratory failure
    B metabolic acidosis and type II respiratory failure
    C metabolic alkalosis and type II respiratory failure
    D mixed respiratory and metabolic acidosis and type II respiratory failure
    E respiratory acidosis and metabolic alkalosis and type I respiratory failure

1.31 A 65-year-old woman was referred because of tiredness, shoulder and hip stiffness and pain, waking her at night persistently for 3 months. Paracetamol gave little relief. She was an insulin dependent diabetic with good control. She had no headache, visual problems, joint swellings or skin rashes.

    On examination she was not in pain. Her pulse was 78 regular and blood pressure 143/88. She had normal tone, power, reflexes and sensation in her limbs. There was normal range of movements and no tenderness was elicited anywhere.

Bloods	Hb	14.4	WCC	6.8
	Platelets	369	ESR	88
	Na	145	K	4.1
	Urea	5.7	Creatinine	100
	Protein	72	Albumin	41
	Bilirubin	8	ALT	20
	ALP	130	GGT	65
	Creatinine kinase	80	Glucose	7.8
	$HbA1_c$	6.9	TSH	1.4
	Free T_4	16		

The most likely diagnosis is:

    A diabetic amyotrophy
    B fibromyalgia
    C giant cell arteritis
    D polymyalgia rheumatica
    E polymyositis

1.32 A 30-year-old woman presented with vaginal discharge and an unpleasant odour post-coitus. She was 18 weeks pregnant with her second pregnancy. The first pregnancy went to term and resulted in a healthy boy being delivered. On speculum examination she produced a thin, watery, homogenous discharge, pH 7.52 (Figure 1.32). See plate section.

Microscopy   No inflammatory cells, no lactobacilli

The most likely diagnosis is:

A bacterial vaginosis
B *Candida sp.*
C *Chlamydia sp*
D *Gonorrhoea sp.*
E *Trichomonas sp.*

1.33 A 23-year-old man presented to Accident & Emergency short of breath (Figure 1.33). See plate section.

Which **ONE** of the following statements is **FALSE**?

A An inspiratory click may be heard on the affected side
B Histiocytosis X could be any underlying cause of his chest problem
C Needle thoracentesis in the second left intercostal space at the midclavicular line should be undertaken
D Pleurodesis should be considered if this problem recurs
E The condition is more prevalent in young, thin men

1.34 A 65-year-old woman presented with early satiety and weight loss (Figure 1.34). See plate section.

The risk factor that is **NOT** associated with her condition is:

A achlorhydria
B alcohol
C blood group O
D *Helicobacter pylori* infection
E smoking

1.35 A 45-year-old woman was admitted with weakness, headaches and palpitations. Her symptoms had been getting worse over the past month. She had no previous medical history. She did not smoke or drink alcohol.

On examination her pulse was 90 regular and blood pressure was 190/105. Her JVP was not elevated and heart sounds and chest examination were normal. Abdominal examination was normal.

Bloods	Na	140	K	2.8
	Urea	5.0	Creatinine	110
	Glucose	6.5	Magnesium	0.65
Arterial blood	pH	7.51	PCO_2	4.5
gases on air	PO_2	11.4	Bicarbonate	35
	Base excess 7.5			

The **LEAST** likely diagnosis in this patient is:

A Conn's syndrome
B Cushing's syndrome
C Liddle's syndrome
D liquorice ingestion
E phaeochromocytoma

1.36 A 55-year-old woman on the intensive care unit had been admitted after an emergency operation for bowel perforation. Now 6 days later she developed worsening shortness of breath. She was no longer being mechanically ventilated. Due to postoperative complications she had been given total parenteral nutrition via a tunnelled central line, which had since been removed. She had no previous medical problems. On examination her pulse was 100 regular and blood pressure 120/84. Her JVP was elevated +4 cm and there was a pansystolic murmur. There were crackles at both lung bases.

Echo   Figure 1.36. See plate section.

The most likely diagnosis is:

A atrial septal defect
B infective endocarditis
C intracardiac thrombus
D myxoma
E ventricular aneurysm

1.37 A 30-year-old woman complained of itching on her hands and forearms for 2 weeks (Figure 1.37). See plate section.

The most appropriate treatment for this patient is:

A oral chlorphenamine (chlorpheniramine)
B oral prednisolone
C topical clotrimazole
D topical hydrocortisone
E topical malathion

1.38 A 56-year-old man was admitted to Accident & Emergency with general lethargy, abdominal discomfort and weight loss. He had been feeling unwell over the last 3 weeks.

Bloods	Calcium 3.22	Phosphate	1.2
	Albumin 35	ALP	120
	PTH 1.0	PTH-related peptide 7.5	

These findings are most consistent with:

    A clear cell carcinoma of the kidney
    B medullary carcinoma of the thyroid
    C oat cell carcinoma of the lung
    D primary hyperparathyroidism
    E tertiary hyperparathyroidism

1.39 It had been proposed that serum CA 19-9 could be used to screen for pancreatic carcinoma. A trial using 600 patients was carried out; of these, 195 cases of carcinoma developed. The CA 19-9 detected 70 cases and 30 false positives. The negative predictive value of CA 19-9 as a screening test is:

    A 70/100
    B 70/195
    C 375/500
    D 375/405
    E 445/600

1.40 A 55-year-old man presented with a distended abdomen that had been getting progressively larger over the past 4 weeks and now caused difficulty with breathing. He admitted to drinking 1 litre of spirits a day for over 10 years.

On examination he was alert and orientated and apyrexial. His pulse was 70 regular and blood pressure 130/80. His chest was clear. His abdomen was tender with shifting dullness.

Bloods	Hb	10.5	WCC	4.8
	Platelets	130	INR	1.0
	Na	130	K	4.3
	Urea	4.5	Creatinine	70
	Albumin	28	Bilirubin	35
	Protein	58	ALT	45
	ALP	120		

The next step in this patient's management would be:

A fluid restrict and institute salt-free diet
B intravenous frusemide
C oral spironolactone
D paracentesis with albumin cover
E transjugular intrahepatic portosystemic stent shunt

1.41 A 58-year-old woman was referred because of a burning sensation and weakness in her legs progressing over some months. She had no previous medical problems and was not on any medication.

On examination her back and legs showed no deformity. There was bilateral lower limb weakness. Tone was increased and the knee jerks were brisk. The ankle jerks were absent and plantars responses were extensor. There was decreased light touch, vibration sense and proprioception. Heel–shin coordination was normal. She walked with a stamping gait and Romberg's test was positive. The most likely diagnosis is:

A Friedreich's ataxia
B motor neurone disease
C multiple sclerosis
D subacute combined degeneration of the cord
E tabes dorsalis

1.42 A 15-year-old girl was admitted with difficulty in breathing. She had had a number of admissions in the past 2 years with the same problem, which had responded to antibiotics. She had a chronic cough, which produced thick yellow sputum. She had no other medical problems. Her current medication included salbutamol nebulisers, aminophylline and oral prednisolone when her breathing got very bad. She did not smoke or drink alcohol. She did not keep any pets and she lived in the middle of town.

On examination her temperature was 37.6°C, pulse 98 regular, blood pressure 100/68 and respiratory rate 22 breaths/min. She had bilateral wheeze plus crackles in the right lower zone of her chest. Abdominal examination was normal.

Bloods				
Hb	12.9	WCC	11.0
Neutrophils	6.3	Lymphocytes	3.5
Eosinophils	1.2	Platelets	250
Na	146	K	4.3
Urea	3.8	Creatinine	67
Protein	76	Albumin	40
Bilirubin	10	ALT	24
ALP	400		

Chest X-ray Patchy shadowing in the right middle and lower lobe
Basal atelectasis on right

The **ONE** feature that would be **LEAST** likely to be consistent with her condition is:

    A elevated serum IgE
    B proximal bronchiectasis on imaging
    C restrictive pattern lung function tests
    D serum precipitins to *Aspergillus* antigen
    E sputum eosinophilia

1.43 A 48-year-old man was referred with a 3-month history of worsening pain in both legs. The pain came on at rest and kept him awake at night. His symptoms were worse in cold weather. He had tried changing shoes with little effect. He could walk about 25 metres before he had to stop and rest. He had no previous medical history or family history of note. He was on no medication. He had smoked 30 cigarettes per day for over 30 years.

His pulse was 90 regular and blood pressure 140/88. His JVP was not elevated and heart sounds were normal. Respiratory and abdominal examinations were normal. There were no palpable pulses below the femoral arteries. He had normal lower limb tone, power and reflexes and sensation to light touch and pinprick. His legs appeared normal but he felt pain on raising them 30° from the horizontal. He had normal range of movements in all joints.

Bloods	Hb	13.7	WCC	6.9
	Platelets	500	INR	1.0
	Na	139	K	4.6
	Urea	7.8	Creatinine	115
	Protein	70	Albumin	40
	Bilirubin	14	ALT	20
	ALP	60	ESR	20
	CRP	10	Glucose	4.4

Rheumatoid factor	Negative
Antinuclear antibody	Negative
ECG	Normal sinus rhythm

The most likely diagnosis is:

    A microscopic polyangitis
    B peripheral neuropathy
    C polyarteritis nodosa
    D sciatica
    E thromboangiitis obliterans

1.44 This 40-year-old man who suffered from pruritus ani had developed a rash over the past 4 months. It was confined to the areas shown. He had been treated with topical betamethasone with no improvement (Figure 1.44). See plate section.

The most likely diagnosis is:

    A Crohn's disease
    B eczema
    C guttate psoriasis
    D pityriasis versicolor
    E ringworm

1.45 A 36-year-old woman presented with a 2-day history of worsening dry cough and shortness of breath (Figure 1.45). See plate section.

The most significant abnormality is in the:

    A left lower lobe
    B left upper lobe
    C right lower lobe
    D right middle lobe
    E right upper lobe

1.46 A 78-year-old man was admitted having collapsed at home. He was sitting at the kitchen table eating his dinner when he suddenly lost consciousness. He remained unresponsive for about 2 minutes. There was no jerking of his limbs or tongue biting but he was incontinent of urine. After regaining consciousness his skin became flushed temporarily. He could not recall any warning, headache or nausea. He was not on any medication and had no previous medical history. His wife mentioned that this was the third time in 3 weeks this had happened without any warning. He did not drink alcohol or smoke.

    On examination he was well. His temperature was 36.7°C, pulse 42 regular and blood pressure 123/79. His JVP was not elevated and both heart sounds were normal. There were no murmurs, extra sounds or carotid artery bruits. Respiratory examination was normal. Central nervous system examination revealed no abnormality. He had normal tone, power, reflexes and sensation in all limbs. Cerebellar function was intact.

ECG   Sinus bradycardia with rate of 42/min

        No ischaemic changes

The most likely diagnosis is:

    A orthostatic syncope
    B Stokes–Adams syncope
    C temporal lobe epilepsy
    D transient ischaemic attack
    E vasovagal syncope

1.47 A 53-year-old woman was referred because of a 3-month history of blisters occurring all over her body, which started off in her mouth. She had no other medical problems and was not on any medication. The skin surrounding the lesion was fragile and if pressed appeared to come off (Figure 1.47). See plate section.

The most likely diagnosis is:

A bullous pemphigoid
B pemphigus vulgaris
C epidermolysis bullosa
D dermatitis herpetiformis
E scalded skin syndrome

1.48 A 19-year-old woman was referred with a 3-month history of excessive thirst and polyuria. She had no previous medical history but earlier in the year she was involved in a car accident in which she suffered minor injuries. On examination she looked well and no abnormalities could be found. A water deprivation test was arranged:

Time after starting (hours)	Plasma osmolality (mosmol/kg)	Urine osmolality (mosmol/kg)
0	295	110
2	300	115
4	306	122
6	310	127
DDAVP 2 μg given intramuscularly		
8	307	320
Plasma$_{ADH}$ post water deprivation test:	undetectable	

The most likely diagnosis in this patient is:

A complete central diabetes insipidus
B complete nephrogenic diabetes insipidus
C partial central diabetes insipidus
D partial nephrogenic diabetes insipidus
E primary polydipsia

1.49 A 57-year-old man was referred with a 7-month history of diarrhoea, opening his bowels four times a days with loose stools. There was no blood or mucus. There was no associated abdominal pain, nausea or vomiting. A year ago he was diagnosed with asthma and this had been difficult to control. He smoked 10 cigarettes per day and drank 2 units of alcohol in the evening.

On examination he looked plethoric. He was apyrexial, pulse 100 regular and blood pressure 150/95. He had bilateral wheeze and palpable hepatomegaly. Rectal examination was normal.

Bloods	Hb	13.5	WCC	5.8
	Platelets	360	Na	140
	K	4.5	Urea	3.7
	Creatinine	90	Albumin	35
	Protein	72	Bilirubin	15
	ALT	35	ALP	130
	Chloride	75	Bicarbonate	24

The test that would give the definitive diagnosis would be:

A serum gastrin
B serum VIP
C stool laxative screen
D urinary 5-HIAA
E urinary VMA

1.50 A 65-year-old woman presented with back, hip and knee pain of 2 years duration. She was currently taking diclofenac and paracetamol for her symptoms. She had not had any falls in the past. She smoked 20 cigarettes per day for over 40 years and drank 2 units of alcohol per day.

 On examination she was a rather obese. She had tenderness and bony swelling of her distal and proximal interphalangeal joints. There was similar swelling and tenderness but no active inflammation of her knees and hips.

Which **ONE** of the following statements is true about her condition?

A Alcohol is not a predisposing factor
B Early menopause is a predisposing factor
C Her symptoms are likely to improve with exercising of the joints
D Previous trauma is not a predisposing factor
E Steroids should be tried if current treatment is ineffective

1.51 A 69-year-old woman was referred because of painful hands. There had been tenderness and swelling in her hands and fingers for 4 months (Figure 1.51). See plate section.

The most likely diagnosis is:

A gout
B hyperparathyroidism
C Paget's disease of bone
D rheumatoid arthritis
E sarcoidosis

1.52 A 3-year-old girl presented with her parents. They were concerned about bleeding from the lesion on her back (Figure 1.52). See plate section.

Which **ONE** of the following statements concerning her condition is **TRUE**?

A Females are more likely to develop these lesions than males
B The majority of the lesions are not present at birth
C Approximately 5% of these lesions will undergo sarcomatous transformation
D She should undergo laser treatment as her lesion has not resolved
E The lesion is full of serous fluid

1.53 A 30-year-old hypertensive woman was found to have an adrenal mass on CT abdomen. The surgeons wanted to resect the mass as it appeared to be localised purely to the adrenal gland. The anaesthetist has asked you to control her blood pressure preoperatively. Prior to admission she was treated with bendroflumethiazide (bendrofluazide).

Her pulse was 95 and her blood pressure 180/90. Cardiovascular, respiratory and thyroid examinations were normal.

Bloods	Na	138	K	4.3
	Urea	4.9	Creatinine	100
	Glucose	7.5	Bicarbonate 25	

24-hour urinary VMA 60

ECG Sinus tachycardia

Left ventricular hypertrophy

Chest X-ray No evidence of failure

The most appropriate antihypertensive for this patient would be:

A methyldopa
B nifedipine
C phenoxybenzamine
D propranolol
E spironolactone

1.54 A 45-year-old woman presented with a 3-month history of abdominal pain and loose stools, worse after eating meals. Four months ago she had had an uncomplicated laparoscopic cholecystectomy. Her appetite was normal with no weight loss. She had no other medical history and was on no medication. She did not drink alcohol.

On examination she was apyrexial and was not jaundiced. Her pulse was 72 regular and blood pressure 130/75. There was mild upper abdominal tenderness and rectal examination was normal.

Bloods	Bilirubin	15		Albumin	35
	ALT	26		ALP	90
	GGT	50		Amylase	45
	CRP	5		Calcium	2.22

Abdominal Cholecystectomy noted; no gallstones seen
ultrasound No abnormalities of liver, pancreas, spleen, kidneys

The most appropriate treatment would be:

A aluminium hydroxide
B colestyramine
C gluten-free diet
D mebeverine
E prednisolone

1.55 A 19-year-old man was referred because of failure to develop secondary sexual characteristics. He had a cleft palate and was colour blind. He was not on any medication. He was adopted and knew nothing of his family history.

On examination there was no gynaecomastia. He had small, soft testes and normal but small male external genitalia.

Bloods	Testosterone	4	(normal: 10–29 nmol/L)
	FSH	0.5	(normal: 1–7 U/L)
	LH	0.5	(normal: 1–6 U/L)
	Prolactin	100	
	TSH	2	Free T$_4$ 26

MRI pituitary Normal

The most likely karyotype of this patient is:

A 45,XO
B 46,XO
C 46,XY
D 47,XXY
E 47,XYY

1.56 A 50-year-old woman was admitted because of recurrent upper abdominal pain. The pain was worse after eating and could last up to 24 hours. It radiated to the back and there were no relieving factors. She had no previous medical history. She did not drink or smoke.

On examination she was not jaundiced or dehydrated. Her temperature was 37.6°C, pulse 95 regular and blood pressure 130/85. There was diffuse upper abdominal tenderness, no organomegaly and rectal examination was normal.

Bloods

Hb	13.9	WCC	12.5
Platelets	300	INR	1.1
Na	141	K	4.9
Urea	4.5	Creatinine	75
Bilirubin	18	Protein	65
Albumin	38	ALT	250
ALP	145	GGT	90
Amylase	100		

Chest X-ray Normal

Abdominal X-ray Normal

The most likely diagnosis is:

A acute appendicitis
B acute pancreatitis
C biliary colic
D diverticulitis
E peptic ulcer

1.57 A 32-year-old woman presented with a 2-month history of progressive weakness, fatigue and decreased appetite. She also complained of vague abdominal discomfort and nausea. She had three young children at home and felt depressed a lot of the time. Last year Graves' disease was diagnosed, from which she was making a slow recovery. Her mother suffered from type 1 diabetes.

On examination she still had some exophthalmos and a small goitre. Her skin was tanned but there was no jaundice or lymphadenopathy. Her pulse was 90 and her blood pressure was 100/65. Clinically she was euthyroid. Abdominal examination revealed generalised tenderness but no organomegaly or guarding.

Bloods

Hb	12.1	WCC	7.8
Platelets	250	Na	132
K	5.9	Urea	6.7
Creatinine	69	Protein	70
Albumin	39	Bilirubin	15
ALT	26	ALP	110
Calcium	2.34	TSH	2.3
Free T$_4$	35	Glucose	3.2

The most likely diagnosis is:

A MEN I syndrome
B MEN 2A syndrome
C MEN 2B syndrome
D APS I
E APS 2

1.58 A 65-year-old homeless person was brought in looking dishevelled and smelling of alcohol. He was alert and coherent but felt tired. On examination he had poor oral hygiene with gingivitis and bleeding gums. He was not encephalopathic and had a normal gait. The rest of his physical examination was normal.

Bloods   Hb   11.5   WCC   5.7

              Platelets 150   MCV   77.5

The vitamin deficiency he is likely to have is:

A vitamin B_1
B folic acid
C vitamin B_6
D vitamin B_{12}
E vitamin C

1.59 A 66-year-old woman was admitted with an anterior MI for which she received thrombolysis. The next day she became very short of breath but had no chest pain or palpitations. Her medication included aspirin, simvastatin and atenolol.

   Her temperature was 37.0°, pulse 80 regular and blood pressure 75/40. Her JVP was +8 cm and heart sounds were difficult to hear. There was dullness in both lung bases and the respiratory rate was 24 breaths/min.

ECG   Normal sinus rhythm

           Q waves and T wave inversion in V_{1-6}

Echocardiogram   (4 chamber). Figure 1.59. See plate section.

The most likely explanation for her deterioration is:

A acute mitral regurgitation
B dissection of thoracic aorta
C pericardial effusion
D right ventricular infarction
E rupture of interventricular septum

1.60 A 30-year-old man presented with lethargy and malaise 2 days after starting chemotherapy for non-Hodgkin's lymphoma. He had mild abdominal discomfort but had not passed much urine despite drinking plenty.

On examination his temperature was 37.0°C, pulse 95 regular and blood pressure 140/78. His JVP was not elevated and heart sounds and chest were normal. The abdomen was soft and not tender with hepatosplenomegaly but no palpable bladder. Rectal examination was normal. Despite being catheterised he had only passed 200 mL of urine over the preceeding 8 hours.

Bloods				
	Hb	13.5	WCC	10.2
	Platelets	345	Na	130
	K	6.1	Urea	38.5
	Creatinine	450	Protein	65
	Albumin	35	Bilirubin	10
	ALT	35	ALP	130
	Calcium	2.0	Phosphate	2.0

Urinanalysis Red cells 2+, granular casts

The prophylactic medication this patient should have received is:

  A allopurinol
  B furosemide (frusemide)
  C gentamicin
  D sodium bicarbonate
  E methylprednisolone

Answers

1.1 **C**** This is a patient with severe congestive cardiac failure that is getting worse. His condition would be classified as New York Health Association Grade IV failure, as dyspnoea is occurring at rest. He needs intensification of his medication. The best treatment would be adding low dose spirono-lactone. The evidence for this comes from the RALES study.

Pitt B., Zannad F., Remme WJ., et al. (1999) The effect of spironolactone on morbidity and mortality in patients with severe heart failure. Randomized Aldactone Evaluation Study Investigators. *N Engl J Med* **341(10)**:709–17.

1.2 **E*** The ECG shows right bundle branch block (RBBB) with a QRS complex >0.12 s and second R wave in V_2. Left anterior fasicular block is shown by the presence of left axis deviation and an initial R wave in II, III and aVF. With left posterior fasicular block there is RBBB and right axis deviation. With trifasicular block there would also be a prolonged PR interval.

1.3 **A**** Indications for haemodialysis in salicylate overdoses include: plasma salicylate concentrations >700 mg/L; renal failure; pulmonary oedema; convulsions and central nervous system effects not resolved by correction of acidosis; and worsening metabolic acidosis. Delayed gastric lavage could be contemplated for up to 12 hours, as it is possible that not all the pills might have been absorbed. Forced alkaline diuresis should not be used because it does not enhance salicylate excretion and may cause pulmonary oedema. Drug overdoses that can be treated with haemodialysis can be remembered using the mnemonic BLAST: Barbiturates, Lithium, Alcohol (including methanol and ethylene glycol), Salicylates and Theophylline.

1.4 **B*** This boy presents with primary herpetic gingivostomatitis. Erosions, blisters and superficial ulcers can develop, with the clinical picture usually settling within 7–14 days. Systemic aciclovir is used for severe herpetic stomatitis.

1.5 **B**** A middle-aged woman with a malabsorptive disease complains of muscle pains and difficulty in walking. She has osteomalacia shown by low serum calcium and phosphate and high ALP. Diabetic amyotrophy presents with painful wasting of the thigh muscles with loss of knee reflexes. Here there is weakness but no wasting of the quadriceps. With osteoporosis there is no biochemical derangement. Periodic paralysis is associated with hyper-thyroidism and hyperkalaemia.

1.6 **C**** The study design needed is one that will allow us to comment on prognosis. Cohort studies involve choosing a group of patients and following them up over a period of time to see if they develop the disease or not. Case control study could be employed but does not allow causality to be proved and so is not the most appropriate study design in this situation. If mass drop out of subjects was an issue then for practical purposes case control study could be employed.

1.7 **B*** This woman is at risk of osteoporosis because she has had frequent courses of steroids. The T-score compares the patient's bone mass with that of a normal young adult gender- and ethnicity-matched population. Using the World Health Organization scoring system, −1.0 means that the patient has a bone mass that is 1 standard deviation below that of the young reference population. The T score indicates whether or not a patient has osteoporosis. A T score of −1.0 or above is normal; between −1.0 and −2.5 means osteopenia; and below −2.5 means osteoporosis. The Z score compares the patient's bone mass with that of an age-, gender- and ethnicity-matched reference population. The Z score gives an indication of whether or not the bone mass is appropriate for the patient's age. A Z score below −2.0 suggests that there maybe a secondary cause for the bone loss, such as malabsorption, vitamin D deficiency or use of certain drugs like steroids.

1.8 **D***** A young teenager presents with bruising. He is recovering from a viral illness and his full blood count shows thrombocytopenia and a mild lymphocytosis. The bruising is due to the low platelet count. In acute leukaemia one would expect a much higher white cell count and the blood film would show blasts. HSP is a vasculitis that is associated with abnormal platelets but there is no significant drop in the platelet count. HSP, like ITP, can occur following a viral infection. There is no evidence of bone marrow failure as the haemoglobin is normal, making aplastic anaemia unlikely.

1.9 **C*** A patient presents with chronic recurrent abdominal pain that often resolves spontaneously and is normal at laparoscopy. Her mother has similar problems, suggesting an inherited component. This condition would be consistent with hereditary angioedema. Patients may present with abdominal pain due to visceral oedema, severe bronchospasm or with facial angioedema, which does not respond to antihistamines. There are low/deficient levels of C1 esterase inhibitor as well as low C2 and C4. Acute treatment is with C1 esterase inhibitor or fresh frozen plasma. Long-term treatment is with danazol or α-aminocaproic acid, an inhibitor of plasmin. Acute intermittent porphyria could present similarly to this but some disturbance in the blood results would be expected, such as hyponatraemia, which would imply syndrome of inappropriate ADH secretion. Wiskott-Aldrich syndrome is an X-linked T and B cell disorder associated with eczema, thrombocytopaenia and lymphopaenia.

1.10 **E**** The history is of a patient with COPD treated with antibiotics who now presents with diarrhoea. The other options are possible but the histology shows the characteristic 'volcano' lesion of pseudomembranous colitis.

1.11 D** This patient has a persistent pyrexia, cough, altered bowel habit and abdominal pain without jaundice, which are all characteristic of typhoid. Rose spots tend not to develop until the second week of the illness. None of the other options are associated with cough or sore throat. Dengue and yellow fever are viral haemorrhagic fever, so jaundice and evidence of bleeding would be expected. Malaria must always be excluded in a patient with pyrexia who has been abroad. Malaria is associated with a low/normal neutrophil count but to develop blackwater fever one would expect a low platelet count suggestive of haemolysis. Amoebic dysentery is usually associated with an increased neutrophil count.

1.12 D* In a young lady with chronic headaches, blurred vision, papilloedema and taking the contraceptive pill the most likely diagnosis is benign intracranial hypertension. CT brain shows no evidence of intracranial lesion, which would have to be excluded in a patient with papilloedema. Lumbar puncture with an opening pressure of $40\,cmH_2O$ or more can confirm benign intracranial hypertension. The aim would be to aspirate CSF not only for analysis but also to reduce the intracranial pressure. Treatments include acetazolamide and even repeat lumbar puncture to reduce the intracranial pressure. Blindness may occur through compression of the optic nerve and so visual field testing is necessary. Magnetic resonance venography is the correct answer because a differential diagnosis for benign intracranial hypertension is sagittal vein thrombosis, which may not be detected by CT brain and could give a raised opening pressure as well.

1.13 C** This patient has diabetic maculopathy. There is a circinate of hard exudates in the macular area close to the centre. This implies there may be leakage of fluid affecting the centre of the macula. The patient may require laser treatment.

1.14 C* Using the modified Dukes' classification: Dukes' A colorectal carcinoma is limited to the mucosa; B_1 extends into the muscularis propria; B_2 extends into the serosa; C_1 has 1–4 regional lymph nodes involved; C_2 has >4 regional lymph nodes involved; and D involves distant metastases.

1.15 B** This middle-aged man presents with an acute monoarthritis. The main differential diagnoses are either sepsis or crystal deposition disease, given the speed of onset. An acute hot, swollen, erythematous joint should be assumed to be infected until proven otherwise but there is nothing to suggest that this patient has a bacterial septic arthritis. He has crystals that show negative birefringence to polarised light and would look needle-shaped. Pseudogout crystals are rhomboid-shaped and show positive birefringence. Serum urate may be normal in up to 30% of patients during an acute attack.

1.16 B** This patient has bacterial meningitis until proven otherwise. The most likely organisms are *Neisseria meningitidis* or *Streptococcus pneumoniae*.

Diagnostic tests that need to be taken include blood cultures, nasal and throat swabs for *N. meningitidis* carriage, and serology for *N.meningitidis* and CSF for Gram stain. High dose intravenous antibiotics should not be delayed. Contact tracing is essential to ensure that close contacts are given antibiotic prophylaxis. There is nothing to suggest she has encephalitis.

1.17 B** The CT scan shows a left posterior extradural haematoma most probably due to trauma to the middle meningeal artery. There is a potential space between the dura and the skull vault and any haematoma forming here will be convex in shape toward the brain and skull vault; hence the 'bulging' appearance. Compare this with 5.16.

1.18 A*** This barium swallow shows the characteristic 'bird's beak' appearance of a dilated proximal oesophagus tapering distally at the gastro-oesophageal junction.

1.19 D, H, I** While all the drugs listed help in the management of unstable angina, there is no conclusive evidence that these three improve prognosis or reduce the risk of death post-MI. Other drugs, which do not improve prognosis, include magnesium, digoxin and antiarrhythmics such as flecainide or propafenone.

Aspirin. ISIS-2 (Second International Study of Infarct Survival Collaborative Group). (1988) Randomised trial of intravenous streptokinase, oral aspirin, both, or neither among 17,187 cases of suspected acute myocardial infarction: ISIS-2. *Lancet* **2(8607):**349–60.

Clopidogrel. CAPRIE Steering Committee (1996) A randomised, blinded, trial of clopidogrel versus aspirin in patients at risk of ischaemic events (CAPRIE). *Lancet* **348(9038):**1329–39.

Low molecular weight heparin. Antman EM, McCabe CH, Gurfinkel EP, *et al.* (1999) Enoxaparin prevents death and cardiac ischemic events in unstable angina/non-Q-wave myocardial infarction. Results of the Thrombolysis In Myocardial Infarction (TIMI) 11B Trial. *Circulation* **100:**1593–1601.

Atenolol. ISIS-1 (1986) Randomised trial of intravenous atenolol among 16,027 cases of suspected acute myocardial infarction: ISIS-1. First International Study of Infarct Survival Collaborative Group. *Lancet* **2(8498):**57–66.

ACE inhibitors. Yusuf S, Sleight P, Pogue J, *et al.* (2000) Effects of an angiotensin-converting-enzyme inhibitor, ramipril, on cardiovascular events in high-risk patients. The Heart Outcomes Prevention Evaluation Study Investigators. *N Engl J Med* **342(3):**145–53.

Simvastatin. Scandinavian Simvastatin Survival Study Group (4S) (1994) Randomised trial of cholesterol lowering in 4444 patients with coronary artery disease. *Lancet* **344:** 1383–89.

N3 polyunsaturated fat fish oils. GISSI-Prevenzione Investigators (1999) Dietary supplementation with n-3 polyunsaturated fatty acids and vitamin E after myocardial infarction: results of the GISSI-Prevenzione trial. *Lancet* **354:**447–55.

1.20 D* All permanent pacemakers are given a code describing their function. The first letter identifies the chamber/chambers being paced: A for atrium, V for ventricle and D for both. The second letter indicates the chamber/chambers whose activity is being sensed: A for atrium, V for ventricle and D for both. The third letter denotes the response to sensed information: I means that pacemaker output is inhibited by a sensed event; T means that stimulation is triggered by a sensed event; and D means that ventricular-sensed events inhibit pacemaker output, whereas atrial-sensed events trigger ventricular stimulation. VVI pacemakers are preferred for patients with complete heart block who are in atrial fibrillation because there are no P waves to trigger a ventricular impulse. As VVI pacemakers have only a single lead they would produce a pacing spike just before the QRS complex if they were working properly; this patient has two spikes before the QRS complex, suggesting he has a DDD pacemaker that is working well and therefore is not responsible for his symptoms. Pyrexia can alter the rate of a pacemaker but not anaemia. More advanced pacemakers can respond to body temperature.

1.21 **C*** Carbon monoxide exerts its toxic effects by binding to haemoglobin, preventing oxygen carriage, causing a left shift of the oxyhaemoglobin dissociation curve so that haemoglobin is less likely to give up oxygen and also by interfering with cytochrome oxidases. Pulse oximeters over-read because they cannot distinguish HbCO from HbO_2. Indications for hyperbaric oxygen therapy include pregnancy, coma, failure to respond to conventional therapy, development of neurological sequelae, and HbCO >40%. PCO_2 is not a determinant of prognosis.

1.22 **A**** This patient has droplet-sized psoriasis papules on her back and extensor surfaces of her elbows, which have developed after a streptococcal infection. Psoriatic lesions are not necessarily associated with pruritus or silvery scales. Pityriasis vesicolor is a superficial, non-inflammatory skin infection caused by the yeast, *Malassezia furfur*; it is characterised by sharply demarcated coffee-brown slightly scaling macules that may coalesce to form irregular forms. Lichen planus consists of small, violaceous flat-topped papules with a lacy white pattern on its surface called Wickham's striae.

1.23 **C**** This pregnant woman has developed thyrotoxicosis. She needs treatment with propylthiouracil. Atenolol should be used with caution in pregnancy and would certainly not control her underlying thyroid disease.

1.24 **D**** NNT (number needed to treat) is the number of patients who would need to be treated with aspirin to prevent one death at the end of 1 year. It is the reciprocal of 1/ARR (absolute risk reduction).

Relative risk of death in aspirin group = 5/1000 = 0.005
Relative risk of death in placebo group = 15/100 = 0.015
ARR = 0.015-0.005 = 0.01
NNT = 1/0.01 = 100

1.25 **B**** All patients with haematemesis require endoscopy but only rarely does this need to occur immediately; in any case, patients need to be stabilised first. There is no evidence that H_2 blockers like ranitidine help; however, there is plenty of evidence that a proton pump inhibitor like omeprazole or pantoprazole may be beneficial. A possible reason for this is that haemostasis is more likely if the environment is as neutral as possible, and this is more likely to be achieved with a proton pump inhibitor. There is actually evidence that a proton pump inhibitor is of benefit even if it is given orally. Terlipressin is the treatment of choice for oesophageal variceal bleed. As there is nothing in the history to suggest varices, management should be aimed at assuming this is an ulcer bleed.

1.26 C* This patient has paroxysmal nocturnal haemoglobinuria, which is a red cell abnormality characterised by the presence of a clone of red cells with an abnormal sensitivity to membrane lysis by complement. Patients may present with aplastic anaemia, myelodysplastic syndromes and acute myeloid leukaemia or with evidence of thombosis like Budd–Chiari syndrome (as in this case), deep vein thrombosis and cerebral vein thrombosis. In Ham's test, complement in the patient's serum is activated by acidification.

1.27 B* The slide shows liver with very small, attenuated hepatocytes that stain pink. The paler pink material in between represents the amyloid. Amyloidosis would also stain with Congo red. With haemochromatosis, the hepatocytes would look normal in size but there would be periportal punctate deposits of haemosiderin pigment which stain with Perl's stain. The hepatocytes would look normal in Wilson's disease but the stain used there is rhodanine. There is not the fibrosis of cirrhosis, and hepatocellular carcinoma is associated with large hepatocytes with big nucleoli.

1.28 A* HAART should be delayed until the CD4 count is <350 or the patient is symptomatic. The viral load does not influence the timing of starting HAART in non-pregnant adults but does influence the type of treatment regimen. Standard HAART consists of three drugs: 2 nucleosides + 1 non-nucleoside or 2 nucleosides + 1 protease inhibitor or 3 nucleosides. The danger of starting HAART too early is that viral resistance may develop and so treatment options will be limited with more advanced disease. Long-term co-trimoxazole is given for *Pneumocystis carinii* pneumonia. AZT can cause bone marrow suppression and so should be avoided in patients who are anaemic.

1.29 D** He has Guillain–Barré syndrome. Such patients can deteriorate quickly and may require intensive care admission, especially if there is respiratory compromise. Factors associated with severe disease include: *Campylobacter jejuni* infection; hypoxia; autonomic neuropathy, including arrhythmias, orthostatic hypotension, hypertension; bulbar involvement; age >40 years; worsening vital capacity (not peak flow); and rapid onset of symptoms.

1.30 A** Arterial blood gases are very easy to interpret if they are approached in a logical fashion. First, decide whether the condition is compensated or not compensated. Second, look at the PCO_2 and see if this is high; if so then there is a respiratory acidosis. Third, assess the bicarbonate to see if this is low, as this would be consistent with a metabolic acidosis. Finally, look at the base excess, the more negative the value, the greater the metabolic acidosis. The PO_2 is not strictly part of the acid–base equation and only gives an indication of hypoxia PO_2 <8.0 kPa. Low PO_2 and low PCO_2 indicates type I respiratory failure and low PO_2 and normal/high PCO_2 indicates type II respiratory failure. Using this approach, this patient has an uncompensated metabolic acidosis with type I respiratory failure. This would be consistent with a salicylate or ethylene glycol overdose.

1.31 D*** Polymyalgia rheumatica is a large blood vessel vasculitis characterised by pain and stiffness in the shoulder and pelvic girdle muscles. While patients may complain of weakness, there often is none on clinical examination. It is associated with patients over 50 years of age and patients usually have high ESRs as well as mildly deranged liver function tests. One third of patients may subsequently develop giant cell (temporal) arteritis. Fibromyalgia is associated with normal blood results and tender points on examination. Polymyositis would result in objective weakness and raised creatinine kinase. Amyotrophy is more common in poorly controlled diabetics and would have associated muscle wasting.

1.32 A* Bacterial vaginosis is typically caused by *Gardnerella vaginalis*, *Bacteroides* sp., *Mobiluncus* sp. and *Mycoplasma hominis*. It has a propensity to affect pregnant women and the type of discharge is characteristic in this patient. It is important to treat as it may cause premature delivery. Trichomonas produces a green, frothy discharge with itching. Chlamydia can produce a watery discharge but tends to affect younger females and results in inflammatory cells being seen. In gonorrhorea, female patients are usually asymptomatic, with no discharge unless they develop pelvic inflammatory disease, and microscopy may reveal lactobacilli. Candidal infections are associated with thick, creamy discharge and itching.

1.33 C*** This patient has a large pneumothorax on the right. If he were in distress and had signs of a tension pneumothorax, needle thoracentesis should be performed as soon as possible but on the side of the pneumothorax. There are a number of causes of secondary pneumothoraces but in any condition that can cause cysts on the lung the cysts may rupture to produce a pneumothorax. Pleurodesis should be considered if the patient develops a second pneumothorax on the same side. Hamman's sign is an inspiratory click sometimes heard in patients with small pneumothoraces.

1.34 C** The barium meal shows a mass in the stomach consistent with gastric carcinoma. Patients with blood group A have an increased risk of gastric carcinoma. *H.pylori* can cause chronic atrophic gastritis and in some patients there is decreased secretion of gastric acid leading to achlorhydria. It is for this reason that symptomatic patients who have *H.pylori* should have eradication treatment.

1.35 E** This middle-aged woman presents with hypokalaemia, metabolic alkalosis, hypertension and hypomagnesaemia. Most patients with Conn's syndrome do not present with any clinical features except hypertension and hypokalaemia. However, Cushing's syndrome due to an oat-cell tumour may not present with Cushingoid features due to the advanced nature of the underlying disease. Liddle's syndrome is a renal tubular defect where there is increased sodium absorption and excessive potassium excretion but with no involvement of the renin–aldosterone system.

1.36 B** The echocardiogram shows a bright irregular mass on the tricuspid valve. This patient has infective endocarditis, probably introduced by the central venous catheter. Myxoma is a tumour that usually arises from the body or wall of the heart. Thrombus would have a darker echogenicity. The ventricle and interatrial septum are normal.

1.37 E** This patient has scabies and the photograph shows the characteristic burrow. The diagnosis is confirmed by identifying the mite microscopically. Treatment is with 0.5% malathion aqueous liquid or 5% permethrin cream. The patient is bathed in the ointment for 24 hours but the itching may take 2–3 weeks to resolve.

1.38 A** This patient has hypercalcaemia of malignancy, as evidenced by the normal PTH level and the elevated PTH-related peptide. PTH-related peptide has a similar homology to PTH and causes bone resorption and inhibition of renal calcium excretion. It is produced by squamous carcinomas involving the lung, head, neck and oesophagus; adenocarcinomas of the kidney, bladder, pancreas, breast and ovary; and clear cell carcinoma of the kidney. PTH-rp is not a sensitive test but is very specific for hypercalcaemia of malignancy.

1.39 C** The negative predictive value is the probability that a patient who tests negative really does not have the condition.

	Pancreatic cancer +	Pancreatic cancer −	
CA 19-9 +	70 (a)	30 (b)	100
CA 19-9 −	125 (c)	375 (d)	500
	195	405	600

Negative predictive value = d/d + c = 375/500 = 0.75

1.40 D** A patient with presumed alcoholic liver disease presents with tense ascites. The most appropriate treatment is to relieve his ascites with therapeutic paracentesis. If he had mild ascites, the plan would be to start oral spironolactone. Fluid restriction is useful if patients are hyponatraemic but it must first be established that they are passing urine adequately, otherwise such actions may cause renal failure. A salt-free diet will not help in the acute situation. The aim should be to drain as much fluid as possible with albumin cover. A typical regimen would be to replace every 2 litres of ascitic fluid drained with 100 mL of 20% albumin or 500 mL 4.5% albumin if the patient was haemodynamically compromised.

1.41 **D**** Subacute combined degeneration of the cord is a consequence of vitamin B_{12} deficiency and results in degeneration of the dorsal columns and corticospinal/pyramidal tracts (causing the extensor plantars) along with demyelination of peripheral nerves (causing the absent ankle jerks). If the burning sensation in the spine and limbs occurs with neck flexion it is a referred to as Lhermitte's sign; it indicates that the cervical spinal cord and sensory tracts are diseased. It may occur in other conditions, such as multiple sclerosis, cervical myelopathy, cervical cord tumours and syringomyelia.

1.42 **C*** The underlying condition in this child is likely to be cystic fibrosis with allergic bronchopulmonary aspergillosis (ABPA). This is an allergic reaction to *Aspergillus fumigatus* that often presents in asthmatics as an eosinophilic pneumonia. It is thought to be a type of hypersensitivity reaction but, unlike other forms of aspergillus infection, this type is not invasive. There is no pathognomonic test for ABPA but presence of all the criteria mentioned in the question would make the diagnosis very likely. ABPA would give an obstructive, not restrictive, lung function abnormality.

1.43 **E**** Thromboangiitis obliterans or Buerger's disease is an inflammatory, obliterative, non-atheromatous vascular disease that affects small and medium-sized blood vessels. Patients are usually middle-aged men who smoke. The diagnosis can be confirmed by arteriography. The history is not suggestive of sciatic nerve damage, which would be associated with normal peripheral pulses and usually be unilateral.

1.44 **E****** This patient has sharply defined red, scaling, pruritic lesions with centrifugal spreading. If this were eczema it ought to respond to topical steroids, but as it is a fungal infection steroids allow the infection to spread.

1.45 **D***** The chest X-ray shows right middle lobe collapse. There is a raised right hemidiaphragm and shadowing of the right lower zone obscuring part of the right heart border. An inhaled foreign body, mucus plug, neoplasm or any cause of consolidation could cause this.

1.46 **B***** Stokes–Adams syncope is usually due to transient asystole or ventricular tachyarrhythmia. Patients typically develop sudden loss of consciousness, with no warning, that improves spontaneously. There is no jerking of limbs, tongue biting or headache, although incontinence does occur occasionally. Vasovagal syncope typically occurs in the upright position and is usually preceded by vagally mediated symptoms such as nausea, yawning, sweating or apprehension. Orthostatic syncope is due to hypovolaemia or excessive venous pooling; it tends to occur when adopting the upright position after prolonged bed rest. Apart from the loss of consciousness there is no focal neurological lesion for this to be classed as a transient ischaemic attack.

1.47 A** This patient has blisters all over her body, which have burst to leave red, denuded areas. The bullae also involve mucous membranes, which are characteristic of pemphigus vulgaris; this is very rare in pemphigoid. If the skin next to the vesicles is pressed, the epidermal layers can be removed; this is referred to as Nikolsky's sign and indicates that the keratinocytes within the epidermal tissue have been disturbed by acantholysis. Unlike pemphigoid, there are intercellular deposits of IgG and complement within the epidermis. Pemphigus vulgaris is lethal if left untreated.

1.48 A** Diabetes insipidus is characterised by a low urine osmolality that fails to concentrate with water deprivation. The fact that there is significant concentration of the urine after injection of desmopressin (DDAVP) is consistent with central or hypothalamic diabetes insipidus. This is complete central diabetes insipidus because there is an undetectable level of ADH circulating in the blood even after water deprivation. A plasma osmolality >295–300 mosmol/kg should be an adequate response for the release of ADH. With partial central diabetes insipidus, the kidneys still retain some concentrating ability; the urine osmolality would be expected to be higher than in complete central diabetes insipidus, the expected increase in urine osmolality would be less after DDAVP injection, and there would be reduced but detectable levels of ADH in the blood postdeprivation test. The normal levels of plasma$_{ADH}$ postdeprivation test would be 3–5 pg/mL.

1.49 D*** A patient with bronchospasm, flushing and chronic diarrhoea is most likely to have carcinoid syndrome. The definitive test is a 24 hour urine collection for 5-HIAA.

1.50 A*** This patient has generalised osteoarthritis. Unlike inflammatory arthritides, pain and stiffness of joints is worse with activity, although non-weight bearing exercises like swimming can help. There is no role for oral or parenteral steroids. Predisposing factors for osteoarthritis include advanced age, previous joint trauma, certain occupations (e.g. machine tool operators), abnormal joint mechanics and smoking. Alcohol and early menopause are associated with osteoporosis.

1.51 E** The X-ray shows bone medullary lucency and expansion of the phalanx. There is also some soft tissue swelling. These findings would be consistent with sarcoidosis affecting the hands. Compare this with Figure 4.30.

1.52 B** This young girl has a strawberry naevus, which is a benign haemangioma and full of blood, so potentially it could bleed. The tumour is not present at birth but usually appears within the first month of life. Most tumours start to involute during the first year and many have fully resolved by age 5–7 years. There is no sex predominance. This lesion would be too large to treat with laser and should be treated conservatively; otherwise surgery and steroids would be the treatment options of choice.

1.53 **C**** This patient is likely to have a phaeochromocytoma (see Question 6.43). Prior to the operation her blood pressure would need to be controlled. She needs α-adrenergic blockade first and then β-blockade, otherwise there will be unopposed α-adrenergic stimulation.

1.54 **B**** This patient has had a cholecystectomy and her symptoms are worse after eating. The history is suggestive of bile salt malabsorption. She would respond best to a bile acid sequestrant like colestyramine. This could be investigated by a SeHCAT scan.

1.55 **C**** This patient has hypogonadotrophic hypogonadism or Kallman's syndrome, as there is also colour blindness and midline facial defects. Such patients may also have anosmia. It can be inherited as an X-linked dominant condition. The basic defect is deficiency of gonadatrophin-releasing hormone from the hypothalamus. Unlike Klinefelter's syndrome there is no abnormality with the chromosomal complement (see 4.51).

1.56 **C**** The history is very suggestive of biliary colic. Peptic ulcer disease is not always associated with eating but is more of a continuous disease rather than episodes of severe abdominal pain.

1.57 **E*** This patient has symptoms of adrenal insufficiency The hyperkalaemia and hypoglycaemia are consistent with this diagnosis. The previous medical history of autoimmune thyroid disease and family history of diabetes suggests that this patient has an APS. APS type 2 is associated with adrenal insufficiency, autoimmune thyroid disease and diabetes type 1. Patients may also suffer from gonadal failure or other autoimmune conditions like coeliac disease, vitiligo, pernicious anaemia, alopecia, Sjögren's syndrome and rheumatoid arthritis.

1.58 **E**** This patient has signs of scurvy (vitamin C) deficiency. Lack of vitamin C is associated with mild iron deficiency anaemia. Wernicke–Korsakoff's syndrome due to thiamine deficiency tends to present with ataxia, ophthalmoplegia, nystagmus, global confusional state and polyneuropathy.

1.59 **C**** The 4-chamber echo shows a dark layer surrounding the heart, suggestive of a large pericardial effusion.

1.60 A* This patient has developed 'tumour lysis syndrome' which is a form of uric acid nephropathy. It is characterised by acute renal failure postchemotherapy, with urine showing red cells and granular casts. In lymphoproliferative and myeloproliferative disorders there is increased cell turnover; after starting chemotherapy, massive cell necrosis occurs, leading to increased uric acid production. The uric acid crystals can become deposited in the renal tubules, causing obstruction and acute renal failure. The aim is to prevent the condition from happening by making sure patients are well hydrated and by giving prophylactic allopurinol to block xanthine oxidase in order to prevent hyperuricaemia. Once acute renal failure develops, patients may need dialysis. There is no evidence that prophylactic bicarbonate prevents this complication.

Questions

2.1 A 44-year-old man was admitted to the coronary care unit with an anterior MI. This was his first MI. He was treated with thrombolysis and his chest pain settled. He was a non-insulin dependent diabetic. He had no retinopathy, neuropathy or nephropathy. He was a non-smoker. Current treatment was gliclazide 80 mg b.d. For the first 2 days he was put onto an intravenous infusion of insulin, his blood glucose stick measurements were between 10 and 15. He was now apyrexial, pulse 70 regular and blood pressure 140/80.

Bloods	Glucose	10.9	HbA$_{1c}$	8.5
	Na	140	K	4.5
	Urea	6.7	Creatinine	90

The best way to manage his diabetes currently would be to:

A add metformin to gliclazide
B convert to metformin
C convert to subcutaneous insulin
D increase his dose of gliclazide
E leave him on the current dose of gliclazide

2.2 A 70-year-old man was admitted with an acute coronary syndrome but did not receive thrombolysis. The next day he complained of chest pain and, as the doctor approached the patient to assess him, he collapsed suddenly. He had no pulse and was not breathing. The cardiac monitor next to his bed revealed the following trace:

The next step in the immediate management of this patient would be:

A adrenaline (epinephrine) 1 mg intravenously
B defibrillate 200 J
C lidocaine (lignocaine) 100 mg intravenously
D precordial thump
E start cardiopulmonary chest compressions

2.3 A 42-year-old woman was brought in having collapsed at home. Her husband thought she had taken an overdose a few hours ago but did not know of what. She had a previous medical history of hypertension and depression. She did not drink alcohol.

On examination she was drowsy but could respond to commands. Her temperature was 38.2°C, pulse 120 regular and blood pressure 100/55. Her JVP was not elevated and heart sounds were normal. Respiratory and abdominal examination were normal, although she had a palpable bladder. Her pupils were dilated but there were no other cranial nerve abnormalities; power, tone and reflexes were normal.

Bloods	Hb	14.0	WCC	7.9
	Platelets	239	INR	1.0
	Na	140	K	3.9
	Urea	4.6	Creatinine	88
	Protein	70	Albumin	40
	Bilirubin	9	ALT	25
	ALP	76	GGT	29
	Glucose	5.2		
Chest X-ray	Normal			
ECG	Sinus tachycardia			
Arterial blood gases on air	pH	7.39	PCO_2	4.1
	PO_2	10.8	Bicarbonate	23
	Base excess	−1.0		

The most likely drug overdose she has taken is:

A amitriptyline
B atenolol
C lithium
D paracetamol
E salicylate

2.4 A 25-year-old woman returned from Kenya complaining of some itching in her right shin. She spent most of her time on the beach or on safari. She had no other symptoms (Figure 2.4). See plate section.

The most likely organism to cause this is:

A *Ancylostoma braziliense*
B *Ascaris lumbricoides*
C *Borrelia burgdorferi*
D *Treponema pertenue*
E *Trichophyton mentagrophytes*

2.5 A 70-year-old woman was brought in drowsy and confused. Her daughter said that she had been off her food and had vomited several times that day.

She had decreased skin turgor and a furred tongue. Her temperature was 38.2°C, pulse 105 regular and blood pressure 100/55. Her JVP was not elevated and heart sounds were normal. Her chest was clear. There was vague lower abdominal tenderness. She was unable to walk independently.

Bloods	Hb	12.5	WCC	13.4
	Platelets	200	Na	152
	K	4.0	Urea	19.0
	Creatinine	184	Glucose	42
Arterial blood gases on air	pH	7.34	PCO_2	4.6
	PO_2	10.5	Bicarbonate	28

Urine osmolality 300 mosmol/kg

Urinanalysis Protein 2+, glucose 3+, ketones 1+

The most likely diagnosis is:

A Addison's disease
B Cushing's syndrome
C diabetes insipidus
D diabetic ketoacidosis (DKA)
E hyperosmolar non-ketotic state (HONK)

2.6 There is increased serum ammonia in patients with hepatic encephalopathy. It has been suggested that measuring serum ammonia might be a useful screening tool for detecting encephalopathy. You have been asked to design a study to investigate this possibility.

The most appropriate study design would be:

A case control study
B case reports
C cohort study
D cross-sectional study
E randomised control trial

2.7 A 62-year-old man was referred with a 6-week history of weight loss, jaundice, dark urine and pale stools but no abdominal pain. He had no previous medical history. He drank 2 units of alcohol per week and was a non-smoker. He was on no medication and had not had any blood transfusions in the past. His last trip abroad was over 20 years ago.

On examination he was markedly jaundiced and looked thin. He was apyrexial, pulse 78 regular and blood pressure 120/70. His abdomen was soft and non-tender with 3 cm hepatomegaly below the costal margin.

Bloods	Hb	14.2	WCC	10.9
	Platelets	390	INR	1.0
	Na	135	K	4.2
	Urea	4.5	Creatinine	90
	Bilirubin	96	Albumin	30
	Protein	64	AST	60
	ALP	300	GGT	30

Hepatitis A, B, C serology	Negative
Abdominal ultrasound	Mild hepatomegaly – normal echo texture Normal common bile duct; gallbladder empty with no stones seen Dilated intrahepatic ducts

The most helpful investigation that would establish the diagnosis would be:

A anti-mitochondrial antibodies
B CT abdomen and biopsy of any mass
C magnetic resonance cholangiopancreatography
D percutaneous transhepatic cholangiography
E ultrasound-guided liver biopsy

2.8 A 60-year-old man presented with sudden loss of vision in the left eye. Over the past 3 months he had noticed increased lethargy and loss of weight. He had no previous medical history.

On examination his temperature was 37.0°C, pulse 88 regular and blood pressure 145/90. Cardiovascular and respiratory examination were normal. Abdominal examination revealed palpable splenomegaly. Cranial nerve examination was normal. See Fundoscopy (Figure 2.8) in plate section.

Bloods	Hb	8.0	MCV	98
	WCC	8.2	Neutrophils	5.0
	Lymphocytes	3.0	Monocytes	0.2
	Platelets	450	ESR	140
	Protein	84	Albumin	38
Immunoglobulins	IgG	1.9	IgA	1.2
	IgM	39.7		

Skeletal survey   Normal

The most likely diagnosis is:

A chronic myeloid leukaemia
B monoclonal gammopathy of undetermined significance
C multiple myeloma
D myelofibrosis
E Waldenström's macroglobulinaemia

2.9 A 35-year-old HIV-positive man presented with shortness of breath and cough productive of green sputum. He was not on any treatment and had no other medical problems.

CD4   95

Viral load 18,500

His current condition is LEAST likely to be due to:

A Cytomegalovirus
B Haemophilus influenzae
C Histoplasma capsulatum
D Mycobacterium avium intracellulare
E Nocardia asteroides

2.10 A 67-year-old woman was referred with left-sided abdominal pain associated with change in bowel habit over the past 4 months. She opened her bowels 3–5 times per day associated with some mucus and blood. Her appetite was decreased and she had lost some weight. She had no previous medical problems and was on no medication. There was no history of travel abroad.

On examination she was apyrexial, pulse 75 regular and blood pressure 130/98. She had left iliac fossa tenderness but no organomegaly and bowel sounds were present. Flexible sigmoidoscopy was performed and biopsies were taken (Figure 2.10). See plate section.

The most likely diagnosis is:

A Crohn's disease
B ulcerative colitis
C diverticular disease
D colorectal carcinoma
E irritable bowel syndrome

2.11 A 38-year-old man presented with a 10-day history of fever and myalgia and a 3-day history of abdominal pain and watery diarrhoea. He had returned from the Gambia 2 weeks ago. He had no previous medical problems and apart from mefloquine malaria prophylaxis was on no medication.

On examination he was not jaundiced. His temperature was 38.4°C, pulse 100 regular and blood pressure 110/80. His JVP was not elevated and heart sounds were normal. There was dullness at the right lung base. He had 4cm tender hepatomegaly but no splenomegaly. There was no ascites and rectal examination was normal.

Bloods				
	Hb	12.5	WCC	10.2
	Neutrophils	8.7	Lymphocytes	1.3
	Eosinophils	0.2	Platelets	286
	Na	140	K	4.2
	Urea	4.3	Creatinine	86
	Protein	68	Albumin	35
	Bilirubin	12	ALT	30
	ALP	120	CRP	150

Malaria films Negative

Chest X-ray Elevated right hemidiaphragm

The most likely diagnosis is:

A amoebic liver abscess
B hepatitis A
C hydatid cyst
D schistosomiasis
E typhoid

2.12 A 60-year-old man developed right-sided weakness affecting his face and upper limb 8 hours previously at breakfast. His speech became slurred and his right arm became weak, with some recovery of power in his arm when seen by the general practitioner. There was no headache, loss of consciousness or fits. Three years ago while having an operation he was noted to have atrial fibrillation but was on no medication. There was no other significant previous medical history. He did not smoke but drank two units of alcohol per night.

On examination he was fully conscious and alert. His temperature was 36.5°C, pulse 95 irregular and blood pressure was 135/70. There were no murmurs or carotid bruits. There was a slight right facial droop and expressive dysphasia. His gag reflex was intact and he was able to swallow. Fundoscopy was normal. He had normal tone, power, reflexes and sensation in all limbs with flexor plantar responses.

Bloods	Hb	14.5	WCC	6.7
	Platelets	345	Na	140
	K	4.7	Urea	4.6
	Creatinine	78	PT	11.4
	ESR	6	Glucose	5.5

The most appropriate immediate treatment for this patient would be:

A aspirin 300 mg
B dipyridamole 75 mg
C warfarin
D thrombolysis with TPA
E no treatment until CT head is performed

2.13 A 44-year-old woman was referred with vomiting. As part of the examination, fundoscopy was performed (Figure 2.13). See plate section.

The fundoscopic appearance is most likely to be due to:

A central retinal vein occlusion
B choroidal metastases
C choroidoretinitis
D photocoagulation scars
E retinitis pigmentosa

2.14 A 50-year-old man who was a heavy smoker presented with shortness of breath and productive cough.

Arterial blood gases on air	pH	7.21	PCO$_2$	9.8
	PO$_2$	7.7	Bicarbonate	34.5
	Base excess	6.3		

These blood gases show:

A mixed respiratory and metabolic acidosis with type I respiratory failure
B mixed respiratory and metabolic acidosis with type II respiratory failure
C respiratory acidosis but not in respiratory failure
D respiratory acidosis with type I respiratory failure
E respiratory acidosis with type II respiratory failure

2.15 A 55-year-old woman was referred with a 4-month history of back and shoulder pain. There was no history of trauma. Her symptoms mainly affected the neck, back and shoulder muscles with some shoulder joint pain. She had some morning stiffness, but normal appetite and no loss of weight. There was a previous medical history of migraine and severe tiredness. She did not smoke or drink alcohol. She took paracetamol self-medication.

On examination she looked well. Her pulse was 74 regular and blood pressure 132/78. There was full range of movements of all joints, although some muscle tenderness over the spine and shoulders. Power, tone, reflexes and sensation were normal.

Bloods	Hb	14.3	WCC	7.4
	Platelets	332	Na	138
	K	4.9	Urea	5.2
	Creatinine	83	Protein	70
	Albumin	40	Bilirubin	11
	ALT	18	ALP	68
	GGT	30	Creatinine kinase	75
	ESR	12	CRP	4
	TSH	2.5	Free T$_4$	20

Rheumatoid factor   Negative

The most likely diagnosis is:

   A cervical radiculopathy
   B fibromyalgia
   C osteoarthritis
   D polymyalgia rheumatica
   E polymyositis

2.16 This 45-year-old woman was referred with skin bruising (Figure 2.16). See plate section.

The **LEAST** likely diagnosis is:

   A Behçet's syndrome
   B Ehlers–Danlos syndrome
   C Marfan's syndrome
   D osteogenesis imperfecta
   E pseudoxanthoma elasticum

2.17 A 28-year-old woman was referred because of a 5-month history of progressive shortness of breath and pain in her hands and feet (Figure 2.17). See plate section.

The most likely diagnosis is:

A histoplasmosis
B Hodgkin's lymphoma
C sarcoidosis
D systemic lupus erythematosus
E tuberculosis

2.18 A 21-year-old man presented with a 2-month history of back stiffness and diarrhoea (Figure 2.18). See plate section.

Which **ONE** of the following is **NOT** associated with his rheumatological condition?

A Amyloidosis
B Atrioventricular conduction block
C Crohn's disease
D Pulmonary fibrosis
E Scleritis

2.19 A 15-year-old girl was referred for cardiac catheterisation because of progressive shortness of breath.

	Pressure	Normal value	O₂ saturation
	(systolic/diastolic/mmHg)		(%)
Right atrium (mean)	8	0–8	7,5
Right ventricle	28/8	15–30/0–8	76
Pulmonary artery	45/15	15–30/0–8	85
Left atrium (mean)	12	1–10	96
Left ventricle	132/12	100–140/3–12	97
Aorta	135/70	100–140/60–90	97

The most likely diagnosis is:

A atrial septal defect
B coarctation of the aorta
C Fallot's tetralogy
D patent ductus arteriosus
E ventricular septal defect

2.20 A 71-year-old woman was found collapsed at home. She could not remember what happened and complained of some discomfort in her chest, arms and legs. Her pulse was 60 regular and blood pressure 100/62. Chest and abdominal examinations were normal. ECGs were performed before (A, see page 55) and a few hours after (B, see page 56) she was given treatment.

The treatment likely to have changed the ECG appearances is:

A calcium gluconate
B intravenous amiodarone
C intravenous potassium
D rewarming
E thrombolysis with TPA

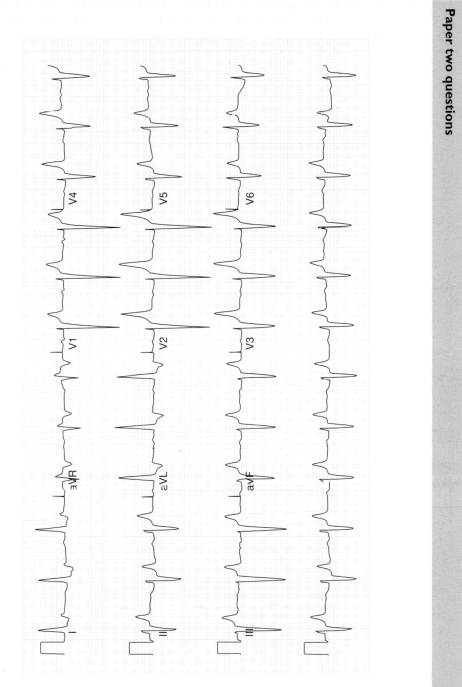

(A)

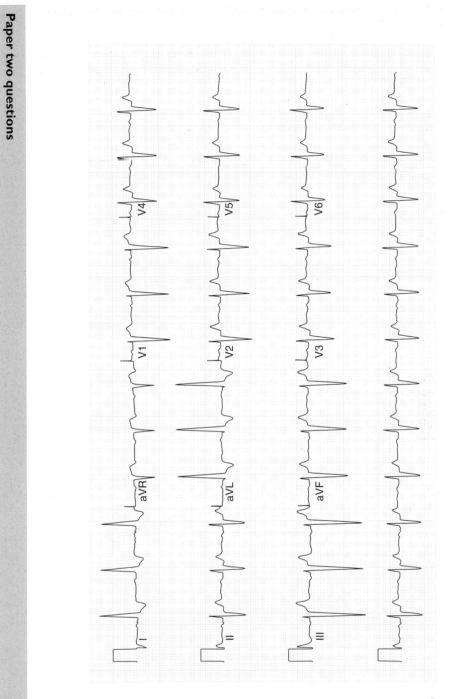

(B)

2.21 A 39-year-old woman known to suffer from depression and schizophrenia was admitted with vomiting, urinary and faecal incontinence and blurred vision. She also had a headache and felt light headed. Her husband thought she had taken an overdose but did not know of what.

On examination she was alert but uncooperative. Her temperature was 36.9°C, pulse 80 regular and blood pressure 100/69. Her JVP was not elevated and heart sounds were normal. Her chest was clear but she had vague abdominal tenderness. She had a tremor at rest and jerky movements of her upper and lower limbs. Her reflexes were brisk and plantar responses were equivocal.

The most likely overdose this patient has taken is:

A amitriptyline
B haloperidol
C lithium
D lorazepam
E propranolol

2.22 A 46-year-old woman with alcoholic liver cirrhosis was referred because of a non-pruritic, blistering rash on her hands, which left scarring. She also complained of increased facial hair growth (Figure 2.22). See plate section.

The most likely diagnosis is:

A bullous pemphigoid
B epidermolysis bullosa
C pemphigus vulgaris
D porphyria cutanea tarda
E scleroderma

2.23 A 55-year-old woman was admitted with central crushing chest pain lasting 2 hours. Her ECG showed atrial fibrillation and T wave inversion in leads II, III and aVF. She was not given thrombolysis. Her pain responded to diamorphine and glyceryl trinitrate.

On examination she was pale but apyrexial. Her pulse was 60 irregular and blood pressure 130/60. Her chest was clear and heart sounds were normal.

Bloods				
Hb	12.5		WCC	9.6
Platelets	270		MCV	86.8
Na	140		K	3.9
Urea	4.7		Creatinine	90
TSH	0.4		Free T$_4$	6

The most likely explanation of these results is:

A primary hyperthyroidism
B primary hypothyroidism
C secondary hypothyroidism
D sick euthyroid syndrome
E surreptitious treatment with thyroxine

2.24 A case control study was performed to see if there was an association between overhead power cables and development of leukaemia. One hundred and sixty subjects were included, of whom 50 patients had leukaemia and 110 control patients did not. Ten leukaemia patients had lived near power cables, as had 30 control patients.

The odds ratio (OR) is:

A $(10 \times 30)/(40 \times 80)$
B $(10 \times 40)/(30 \times 80)$
C $(10 \times 50)/(30 \times 110)$
D $(10 \times 80)/(30 \times 40)$
E $(10 \times 110)/(30 \times 50)$

2.25 A 60-year-old homeless man presented to casualty with confusion. He smelt of alcohol, was verbally abusive but could answer questions.
On examination his GCS was 14/15. He was apyrexial and not jaundiced. His speech was slurred and he was disorientated in time and place but there was no tremor or flap. His pulse was 70 regular and blood pressure 150/100. Chest examination was normal. The abdomen was soft, not tender and mildly distended with shifting dullness. Bowel sounds were present and rectal examination revealed no melaena.

Bloods				
	Hb	12.4	WCC	11.3
	Platelets	100	INR	1.4
	Na	135	K	3.9
	Urea	4.5	Creatinine	56
	Protein	60	Albumin	30
	Bilirubin	20	ALT	55
	ALP	230		

Chest X-ray No abnormality detected

Urinalysis Normal

The next **THREE** steps in his immediate management would be:

A diagnostic ascitic tap
B fresh frozen plasma
C intravenous ranitidine
D intravenous terlipressin
E intravenous thiamine
F intravenous vitamin K
G oral antibiotics
H oral diazepam
I oral lactulose
J oral neomycin
K oral prednisolone
L oral propranolol
M therapeutic paracentesis with albumin cover
N upper gastrointestinal endoscopy

2.26 A 14-year-old boy was referred with a severe nosebleed. He had suffered greatly with nosebleeds in the past; he also tended to bruise easily. He was adopted and knew nothing of his real parents. He was on no medication.

On examination he was apyrexial. He had bruises all over his skin but otherwise there was nothing else to find on physical examination. His nose stopped bleeding spontaneously.

Bloods	Hb	13.5	MCV	78.8
	WCC	5.4	Platelets	155
	APTT	78	PT	13
	TT	20		

APTT with 50:50 mix of normal plasma   44

Bleeding time   16 minutes

Factor VIII 11%

Factor IX   65%

The most likely diagnosis is:

A antiphospholipid syndrome
B circulating antibody to factor VIII
C haemophilia A
D haemophilia B
E Von Willebrand's disease

2.27 A 45-year-old woman was referred with dysphagia and weight loss. There was no haematemesis or melaena. She had no abdominal pain or bowel problems. She smoked 20 cigarettes per day for over 20 years and used to drink 4 units of alcohol per night.

On examination she was not jaundiced or pale. Her pulse was 88 regular and blood pressure 120/69. Respiratory and abdominal examinations were normal. An endoscopy was performed and oesophageal biopsies were taken (Figure 2.27). See plate section.

The most likely diagnosis is:

A Barrett's oesophagus
B normal oesophageal mucosa
C oesophageal candidiasis
D oesophageal adenocarcinoma
E squamous cell carcinoma

2.28 A 19-year-old woman presented with a 5-day history of fever, lethargy and cough followed by abdominal pain and frank haematuria. She had returned from Malawi a week ago where she had been on safari. She had no other medical problems and had taken mefloquine malaria prophylaxis. She had one regular sexual partner and did not drink alcohol or smoke.

Her temperature was 38.0°C, pulse 100 regular and blood pressure 130/80. Physical examination was normal except for some cervical lymphadenopathy.

Bloods	Hb	12.7	WCC	10.8
	Neutrophils	8.4	Lymphocytes	1.4
	Eosinophils	1.0	Platelets	210
	Na	130	K	5.0
	Urea	12.1	Creatinine	200
	Protein	70	Albumin	36
	Bilirubin	10	ALT	28
	ALP	120		

Malaria films Negative

Urinanalysis Protein 1+, blood 3+

Chest X-ray Normal

The most likely diagnosis is:

A blackwater fever
B brucellosis
C dengue haemorrhagic fever
D schistosomiasis
E typhoid

2.29 A 47-year-old man presented with wasting of the muscles of the hand. This problem had developed gradually over the last 12 months. He also had paresthesiae in his hands and feet. He had no problems with vision or speech.

On examination he looked well. There was wasting of the small muscles of the hand with some clawing and decreased pinprick sensation. There was also wasting of the distal lower limb muscles and pes cavus. Dorsiflexion was weak. Tone was normal but the ankle and plantar reflexes were absent. There was decreased pinprick sensation up to the ankle. His gait showed dragging of both feet.

The most likely diagnosis is:

A Charcot–Marie–Tooth disease (HSMN)
B Friedreich's ataxia
C subacute combined degeneration of the cord
D syringomyelia
E tabes dorsalis

2.30 A 21-year-old woman was admitted with shortness of breath of 1 day's duration.

Arterial blood gases on air	pH	7.51	PCO_2	3.1
	PO_2	14.3	Bicarbonate	25
	Base excess	−0.5		

These blood gases show:

A metabolic alkalosis and respiratory acidosis with no respiratory failure
B metabolic alkalosis with no respiratory failure
C mixed respiratory and metabolic alkalosis with no respiratory failure
D respiratory alkalosis and metabolic acidosis with no respiratory failure
F respiratory alkalosis with no respiratory failure

2.31 A 54-year-old man presented with a 6-month history of worsening oedema and shortness of breath on exertion. He had no chest pain but could only manage 10 stairs and became breathless at night sleeping with three pillows. His previous medical history included arthritis affecting wrists, elbows and knees and bilateral carpal tunnel syndrome. He was on furosemide (frusemide). He did not smoke or drink alcohol.

On examination he had pitting oedema up to the sacrum with some facial puffiness and a large tongue. His pulse was 88 regular and blood pressure 160/90. His JVP was elevated to +6 cm and both heart sounds were normal. There was decreased air entry at both bases. His abdomen was distended with shifting dullness and 4 cm hepatomegaly. Apart from wasting of both thenar eminences and paresthesiae in the median nerve distribution of the hands, neurological examination was normal.

Bloods	Hb	11.8	MCV	96.2
	WC	4.9	Platelets	248
	Na	138	K	4.7
	Urea	14.5	Creatinine	170
	Protein	58	Albumin	29
	Bilirubin	18	ALT	35
	ALP	60	Calcium	1.98
	Glucose	5.6	ESR	45
	CRP	30	Vitamin B$_{12}$	210
	Folate	5		

Urine dipstick   Protein   3+

Chest X-ray   Enlarged heart with upper lobe blood diversion

Echocardiogram   Thickened and hypokinetic interventricular septum

The most likely diagnosis is:

   A analgesic nephropathy
   B carcinoid syndrome
   C constrictive pericarditis
   D hypertrophic obstructive cardiomyopathy
   E primary amyloidosis

2.32 This 69-year-old woman was referred because of lethargy. As part of the examination, the following was seen in her mouth (Figure 2.32). See plate section.

The clinical findings would be most consistent with:

   A acromegaly
   B amyloidosis
   C hypothyroidism
   D vitamin B$_{12}$ deficiency
   E vitamin C deficiency

2.33 A 57-year-old woman presented with a 6-week history of progressive dysphagia and weight loss (Figure 2.33). See plate section.

The most likely diagnosis is:

   A achalasia
   B benign stricture due to gastro-oesophageal reflux disease
   C carcinoma of the oesophagus
   D oesophageal candidiasis
   E oesophageal varices

2.34 A 44-year-old woman was referred with a 3-day history of worsening headache, photophobia, nausea and confusion. There was no rash. She had no other medical problems and was not on any medication. She was allergic to penicillin.

On examination she was unwell. Her temperature was 38.1°C, pulse 98 regular and blood pressure 100/60. She was disorientated in time and place but not in person. She had poor short-term memory and her mental test score was 1/10. Kernig's sign was negative. There were no focal neurological signs and plantar responses were flexor.

Bloods	Hb	13.7	WCC	11.0
	Platelets	170	Na	135
	K	4.1	Urea	8.4
	Creatinine	100	Glucose	4.5
	INR	1.2		
CSF	RBC	50	WCC	30
	Neutrophils	45%	Lymphocytes	45%
	Protein	0.8	Glucose	3.1

MRI scan Figure 2.34. See plate section.

The most appropriate drug treatment for this patient is:

A aciclovir
B cefotaxime
C chloramphenicol
D pyrimethamine and sulfadiazine
E rifampicin, isoniazid and pyrazinamide

2.35 A 59-year-old woman was admitted with pleuritic chest pain and pyrexia. She had no cough, shortness of breath or leg swelling. Four weeks ago she suffered an anterior myocardial infarction, treated with thrombolysis, and had made an uneventful recovery. She had no other previous medical problems. She was taking, since discharge: aspirin, atenolol, simvastatin and isosorbide mononitrate. She did not smoke or drink alcohol.

On examination she was not in pain. Her temperature was 37.6°C, pulse 72 regular and blood pressure 110/70. Her JVP was not elevated. There was an additional heart sound but no murmurs. Her chest was clear. Examination of both lower limbs was normal.

Bloods	Hb	13.0	WCC	11.0
	Platelets	368	INR	1.1
	Na	138	K	4.5
	Urea	4.2	Creatinine	88
	ESR	32	CRP	28

ECG	Q waves in V_{2-6}		
	Minimal ST elevation in V_{2-6} unchanged when compared to previous ECGs		

Arterial blood gas on air	pH	7.43	PCO_2	4.3
	PO_2	11.3	Bicarbonate	25.4
	Base excess	1.1		

The most appropriate treatment for this patient is:

A amoxicillin
B diclofenac
C furosemide (frusemide)
D nicorandil
E warfarin

2.36 A 64-year-old man was admitted with palpitations and collapse. He had a previous medical history of hypertension but was not on any medication. He did not drink alcohol or smoke. His temperature was 37.3°C and blood pressure 110/68.

The ECG shows:

A atrial fibrillation with aberrant conduction
B supraventricular tachycardia with aberrant conduction
C torsades de pointes
D ventricular fibrillation
E ventricular tachycardia

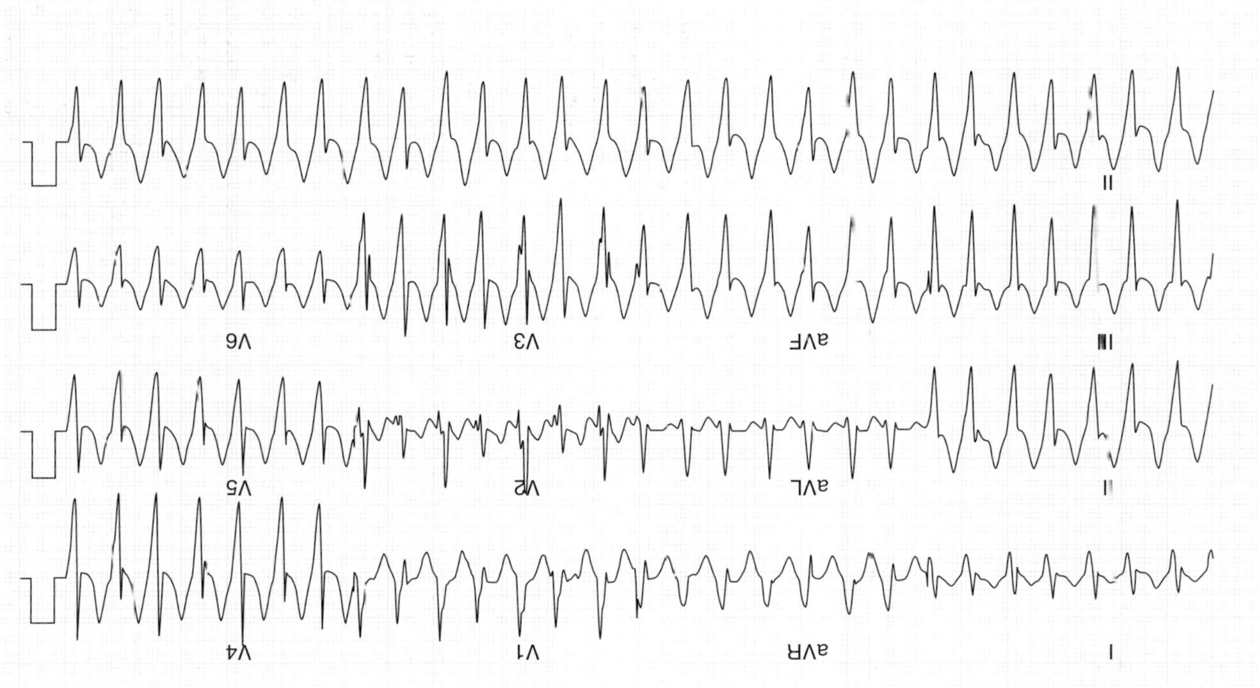
I
aVR
V1
V4
II
aVL
V2
V5
III
aVF
V3
V6
II

2.37 A 42-year-old man was referred with a 3-week history of an ulcerating lesion on his left leg. He was not on any medication (Figure 2.37). See plate section.

Which **THREE** of the following conditions are **NOT** associated with this skin lesion?

A Acute myeloid leukaemia
B Ankylosing spondylitis
C Carcinoid syndrome
D Crohn's disease
E Polycythaemia rubra vera
F Porphyria cutanea tarda
G Rheumatoid arthritis
H Sarcoidosis
I Tuberculosis
J Tuberous sclerosis
K Ulcerative colitis
L Wegener's granulomatosis

2.38 An 18-year-old man with learning difficulties presented with numbness and muscle cramps.

Bloods	Calcium	1.95	Phosphate	1.6
	Albumin	40	ALP	100
	PTH	7.0	25-Vitamin D$_3$	75
	1,25-Vitamin D$_3$	45		

These blood results are most consistent with:

A cirrhosis
B hypomagnesemia
C hypoparathyroidism
D pseudohypoparathyroidism
E pseudopseudohypoparathyroidism

2.39 A 55-year-old female Jehovah's Witness was found to have a carcinoma of the colon at colonoscopy. The colorectal surgeon recommended a total colectomy but informed the patient that this would incur substantial blood loss. The patient was adamant that she did not want a 'blood transfusion', even if she were to exsanguinate on the operating table.

Which **ONE** of the following would be acceptable to her for the surgeon to perform the operation?

A Fresh frozen plasma
B Intraoperative autotransfusion of blood collected during operation
C Packed red cells
D Platelet transfusion
E Predonation of her own blood with autologous transfusion if necessary

2.40 A 23-year-old woman was referred with a 6-month history of weight loss and abdominal discomfort. Her symptoms were worse if she ate wheat. She had no other medical problems and was on no medication. Physical examination was entirely normal. A possible diagnosis of coeliac disease was contemplated.

Which **ONE** of the following concerning the diagnosis of coeliac disease is **FALSE**?

A After starting a gluten-free diet she should have a repeat endoscopy to ensure healing
B Histology will show crypt abscesses
C If the patient has IgA deficiency antigliadin and antiendomyseal antibodies may be negative even if she has coeliac disease
D She may have a dimorphic blood film
E Tissue transglutaminase is a specific test for coeliac disease

2.41 A 29-year-old woman was admitted with palpitations. She had no previous medical history. She did not drink or smoke and was not on any medication.

Which **ONE** of the following drugs should be avoided with her condition?

A Adenosine
B Amiodarone
C Flecainide
D Sotalol
E Verapamil

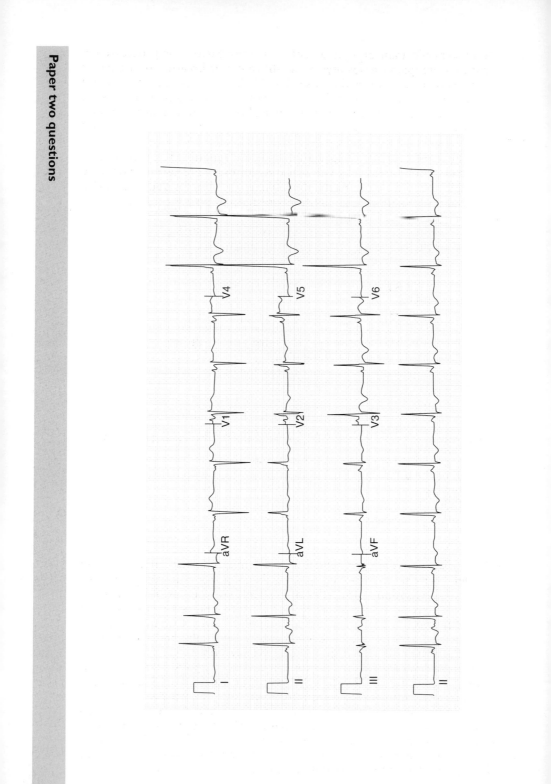

2.42 A 28-year-old man presented with a 1-week history of progressively worse haemoptysis associated with shortness of breath. Subsequently he had passed frank blood in his urine. He had no bowel problems and there was no abdominal pain or haematemesis. He had no joint or skin problems. There was no previous medical history or significant family history. He smoked 20 cigarettes per day and drank 4 units of alcohol at the weekend.

On examination his temperature was 37.3°C, pulse 110 regular and blood pressure 115/80. His JVP was not elevated and heart sounds were normal. There was decreased air entry at his lung bases but no crackles or wheeze. Abdominal examination was normal.

Bloods	Hb	11.5	MCV	80.1
	WCC	9.6	Platelets	245
	Na	135	K	6.3
	Urea	32.4	Creatinine	452
	Protein	70	Albumin	32
	Bilirubin	15	ALT	28
	ALP	65	Calcium	2.24

Urine dipstick Protein 2+, blood 3+

Chest X-ray Bilateral patchy densities

The blood test that would be most helpful in establishing the diagnosis is:

A anti-glomerular basement membrane antibodies
B antinuclear antibodies
C p-ANCA
D rheumatoid factor
E serum cryoglobulins

2.43 A 47-year-old woman presented with a 1-month history of an ulcer on her left shin that did not appear to be healing. She also complained of decreased sensation in the soles of her feet. For the past 6 months she had been having recurrent attacks of sinusitis and epsistaxis. She had now developed a cough associated with blood-tinged sputum. She had a decreased appetite and had lost some weight. She had no previous medical history. She did not smoke or drink alcohol.

On examination her temperature was 37.6°C, pulse 78 regular and blood pressure 157/79. Her JVP was not elevated and both heart sounds were normal. Her respiratory rate was 20 breaths per minute and she had bilateral crackles in her chest. Abdominal examination was normal. There was a 3 cm ulcer on her left shin that appeared 'punched out' with surrounding erythema. She had decreased sensation to light touch and pinprick up to the level of the ankles. There was normal lower limb tone and power but absent ankle and plantar reflexes.

Bloods	Hb	11.9	MCV	92.4
	WCC	7.6	Platelets	459
	Na	138	K	4.8
	Urea	12.4	Creatinine	150
	Protein	74	Albumin	38
	Bilirubin	15	ALT	55
	ALP	100	ESR	65
	CRP	58	C3	100
	C4	35		

Rheumatoid factor   Negative

Antinuclear antibody   Negative

Hepatitis A, B and C serology   Negative

Urine dipstick   Blood 2+, protein 3+, red cell casts +

Chest X-ray   Bilateral infiltrates

No consolidation, no pulmonary oedema

The most likely diagnosis is:

    A Goodpasture's syndrome
    B mixed cryoglobulinaemia
    C polyarteritis nodosa
    D systemic lupus erythematosus
    E Wegener's granulomatosis

2.44 A 72-year-old man complained of headaches. He also had pain in his back and hips (Figure 2.44). See plate section.

The most likely diagnosis is:

    A acoustic neuroma
    B hypoparathyroidism
    C metastatic lung carcinoma
    D multiple myeloma
    E Paget's disease of bone

2.45 A 58-year-old woman was referred with ulceration of her right index finger (Figure 2.45). See plate section.

The most likely diagnosis is:

A rheumatoid arthritis
B psoriatic arthropathy
C dermatomyositis
D systemic sclerosis
E systemic lupus erythematosus

2.46 A 49-year-old women presented with weakness affecting all her muscles, including those of her face. This problem had been getting progressively worse over several years. She had also noticed some slurring of her speech. Recently she had been found to have diabetes mellitus. She smoked 20 cigarettes per day for thirty years.

On examination she had a left ptosis. There was wasting of her facial, temporalis, sternocleidomastoid, shoulder and quadriceps muscles. She had normal tone but reduced power and reflexes. She had difficulty opening her eyes. Sensation and gait were normal. Cardiovascular and respiratory systems were normal. The most likely diagnosis is:

A dystrophia myotonica
B myasthenia gravis
C Eaton–Lambert syndrome
D motor neurone disease
E diabetic amyotrophy

2.47 A 65-year-old homeless man was brought to Accident & Emergency suffering from self-neglect. He denied any medical problems and was not on any medication.

He was alert and orientated but appeared obviously cachexic and dehydrated. The rest of the physical examination was normal.

It was decided to give him intravenous dextrose, insert nasogastric tube and feed him via this route.

Three days later, he became acutely short of breath and very oedematous. His temperature was 37.2°C, pulse 110 regular and blood pressure 140/80. JVP was elevated to +6 cm and he had bilateral crackles in his chest.

Bloods				
Hb	12.5	WCC	6.8
Platelets	245	Na	132
K	2.9	Urea	6.4
Creatinine	58	Albumin	24
Protein	50	Bilirubin	17
ALT	24	ALP	90
Glucose	4.5	Calcium	1.98
Magnesium	0.65	Phosphate	0.6

The most likely cause for his deterioration is:

A aspiration pneumonia
B fluid overload with intravenous dextrose
C kwashiorkor
D protein-losing enteropathy
E refeeding syndrome

2.48 A 65-year-old man was referred because of worsening tremor and poor mobility. The tremor was so bad he could not hold a cup without spilling the contents. His handwriting was getting progressively smaller.

On examination he had no facial abnormalities. There was increased tone in his upper limbs and an obvious resting tremor that became worse when he was asked to lift an object. He had normal power and reflexes but his gait was shuffling.

The drug treatment that would **NOT** be used to treat his illness is:

A apomorphine
B tetrabenazine
C baclofen
D entacapone
E bromocriptine

2.49 A 72-year-old woman was discharged from hospital after being admitted with an exacerbation of COPD. She had had COPD for 5 years and it was gradually getting worse: she had been admitted four times this year with the same problem. She had salbutamol and ipratropium bromide nebulisers at home and oxygen cylinders to be used on 'as needed' basis. She stopped smoking last year, but prior to that was smoking 30 cigarettes per day for 50 years.

On examination her pulse was 100 regular and blood pressure 145/98. Her JVP was not elevated and both heart sounds were normal. Her respiratory rate was 18 breaths/min and her chest was clear to auscultation.

Arterial blood gases on air	pH	7.35	PCO_2	5.6
	PO_2	7.1	Bicarbonate	38.5
	Base excess	12.4		

Which **ONE** of the following would **NOT** be a determinant in deciding whether this patient needed long-term oxygen therapy?

A Exercise tolerance less than 5 metres
B $FEV_1 \leq 1.5l$
C $PaO_2 \leq 7.3\,kPa$ on air
D $PaO_2 \leq 8.0\,kPa$ on air with evidence of pulmonary hypertension
E Stopping smoking completely

2.50 A 45-year-old woman with Crohn's disease was referred with pain in her left hip for the past 6 weeks. The pain was localised to the buttock, groin, medial thigh and knee and made her walk with an antalgic gait. There was no back pain or stiffness or other joint pains. She had a normal appetite and no weight loss. She did not smoke or drink alcohol. Her current medication was mesalazine and prednisolone and she had had numerous courses of steroids in the past. There was no history of trauma.

On examination she was in pain. Her temperature was 37.0°C, pulse 88 regular and blood pressure 125/88. Respiratory and abdominal examination was normal. The left hip did not appear obviously inflamed but all movements caused severe pain. There was normal sensation and peripheral pulses were all palpable.

Bloods	Hb	13.4	WCC	5.8
	Platelets	260	Na	138
	K	4.0	Urea	4.9
	Creatinine	88	Protein	70
	Albumin	37	Bilirubin	10
	ALT	25	ALP	75
	Calcium	2.20	Phosphate	0.74
	ESR	12	CRP	26

Rheumatoid factor Negative

DEXA scan of total hip T score −0.8

Z score −0.5

The most likely diagnosis is:

A fibromyalgia
B osteoarthritis
C osteomalacia
D osteonecrosis
E osteoporosis

2.51 A 52-year-old female had an MRI scan because of difficulty walking and lack of coordination. She had a normal appetite and no weight loss. She had no previous medical history and was not on any medication. There was no significant family history (Figure 2.51). See plate section.

The scan results would be most consistent with a diagnosis of:

A Huntington's chorea
B metastatic disease
C multiple sclerosis
D normal pressure hydrocephalus
E variant Creutzfeld–Jakob disease

2.52 A 36-year-old woman was referred with a pigmented mole that had increased in size (Figure 2.52). See plate section.

Which **ONE** of the following is associated with a **BETTER** prognosis?

A Less than 15 mm thick
B Less than 4 cm in diameter
C Located in the anorectal region
D Located in the buccal mucosa
E Located on the upper thigh

2.53 A 16-year-old girl presented, with her mother, complaining of primary amenorrhoea. She had been brought up as a girl. She had normal breast development but no axillary or pubic hair. She had no previous medical history and had had a normal development up until now. She was not on any medication.

On examination she was of normal height and weight for her age. Her pulse was 78 and blood pressure 110/70. She had normal breasts. She had normal female external genitalia.

Chromosome analysis	46,XY
Bloods	17-OH Progesterone 7.0 (normal: <10 nmol/L)
	FSH 3.5 (normal: 1–8 U/L)
	LH 10.4 (normal: 1–6 U/L)
Pelvic ultrasound	Absent uterus
	Bilateral undescended testes

The most likely diagnosis is:

A 11-β-hydroxylase deficiency
B androgen insensitivity
C gonadal dysgenesis
D Kallman's syndrome
E Klinefelter's syndrome

2.54 A 55-year-old man was found on barium enema to have a colonic carcinoma affecting the caecum. There was no other mass in his large intestine, and abdominal ultrasound revealed no liver metastases. He had a right hemicolectomy. Histology of the mass revealed poorly differentiated adenocarcinoma with invasion through to the muscularis propria but with five regional lymph nodes invaded. The likely 5-year survival for this patient with treatment would be:

A 20%
B 40%
C 60%
D 75%
E 85%

2.55 A 17-year-old girl was referred with primary amenorrhoea. Since childhood she had had poor growth despite proper care from her parents. Her father was 1.80 m tall and her mother was 1.65 m tall. She had suffered from recurrent urinary tract infections in the past.

On examination she was 1.30 m tall and her weight was 40 kg. There was no breast development and there were no secondary sexual characteristics. The rest of her appearance was normal.

Bloods			
	FSH	40	(normal: 2.5–10 U/L)
	LH	27	(normal: 2.5–10 U/L)
	17-β-oestradiol	45	(normal: 70–370 pmol/L)
	17-OH Progesterone	7	(normal: <14 nmol/L)
	Progesterone	1.5	(normal: <5 nmol/L)
	Prolactin	400	

Pelvic ultrasound Small uterus
Ovaries not seen very well
Duplex kidneys

Which **ONE** of the following statements concerning her likely condition is true?

A As her progesterone level is normal she only needs cyclical oestrogen therapy
B Growth hormone therapy may improve her stature
C In the majority of patients cardiac abnormalities would be expected
D There is an abnormality on chromosome 13
E This is a form of congenital adrenal hyperplasia

2.56 A 48-year-old man presented with a 1-week history of persistent dull upper abdominal pain and fever. He also complained of pale stools and episodic dark urine. He had decreased appetite, some weight loss and looked yellow. Eighteen months earlier he had undergone laparoscopic cholecystectomy for gallstones, and ERCP 4 months ago to remove sludge from the common bile duct. He drank 10 units of alcohol per week and smoked 15 cigarettes per day. He was not on any medication.

On examination he was jaundiced, had a temperature of 39.1°C, pulse 120 regular and blood pressure 120/60. There was right upper quadrant abdominal tenderness but no hepatosplenomegaly and no ascites. Rectal examination was normal. He was not encephalopathic.

Bloods				
	Hb	12.5	WCC	15.6
	Platelets	345	INR	1.5
	Na	136	K	4.5
	Urea	5.9	Creatinine	120

Bilirubin	62	Albumin	30
Protein	60	AST	60
ALP	360	GGT	140

Chest X-ray Normal

Urinalysis Bilirubin 1+, no protein, no white cells

The most likely diagnosis is:

A ascending cholangitis
B cholangiocarcinoma
C primary biliary cirrhosis
D primary sclerosing cholangitis
E secondary biliary cirrhosis

2.57 A 57-year-old man was referred with severe abdominal pain, worse after eating but no vomiting. Three months ago a duodenal ulcer had been diagnosed and a proton pump inhibitor started but his symptoms had returned. He had decreased appetite and had lost some weight. He also complained of watery diarrhoea, which woke him from sleep. He was on no other medication.

On examination there were no abnormal findings apart from epigastric tenderness. He was admitted for investigation, all medication having been stopped.

Bloods	Hb	10.5	WCC	5.6
	Platelets	450	Na	140
	K	4.3	Urea	5.5
	Creatinine	79	Chloride	100
	Amylase	120	Calcium	2.24
	Albumin	39		

Fasting serum gastrin	250
Serum gastrin after secretin infusion	340
Repeat upper GI endoscopy	Two chronic duodenal ulcers
CT abdomen	Mass arising from pancreas

The most likely diagnosis is:

A gastrinoma
B glucagonoma
C insulinoma
D somatostatinoma
E VIPoma

2.58 A 55-year-old Bangladeshi woman was treated for pulmonary tuberculosis (TB). She was started on rifampicin, isoniazid, ethambutol and pyrazinamide. After 2 months of treatment she complained of tingling in her fingers.

On examination she had sensory loss in a glove distribution in both upper limbs up to the level of the metacarpophalangeal joints and in a stocking distribution up to her ankles. She had no loss of power, tone or reflexes. She also had some glossitis.

The vitamin deficiency she is likely to have is:

A vitamin B_1
B vitamin B_2
C vitamin B_6
D vitamin B_{12}
E vitamin C

2.59 A 38-year-old man was referred because of repeated episodes of chest pain and shortness of breath.

On examination his pulse was 80 regular and blood pressure 126/80. His JVP was not elevated and there was a loud systolic murmur. His chest was clear.

Echocardiogram   Figure 2.59. See plate section.

The most likely diagnosis is:

A aortic stenosis
B atrial septal defect
C hypertrophic obstructive cardiomyopathy
D myxoma
E ventricular septal defect

2.60 A 70-year-old woman on the orthopaedic ward developed oliguria 10 days after an emergency operation for a fractured neck of femur. She had a previous medical history of osteoarthritis. She was on diclofenac. She had been receiving intravenous fluids and cefuroxime and gentamicin postoperatively.

On examination she had minimal ankle oedema. She was apyrexial, pulse 95 regular and blood pressure 120/80. JVP was elevated to +2 cm and she had a soft third heart sound. Breath sounds were decreased at both lung bases. Her abdomen was soft with no organomegaly. She had passed 100 mL of urine in the preceding 12 hours.

Bloods				
Hb	12.9	WCC	10.5
Platelets	360	Na	135
K	6.5	Urea	50.1
Creatinine	1100	Protein	66
Albumin	35	Bilirubin	11
ALT	23	ALP	110
Calcium	2.22	Phosphate	2.1

Arterial blood gases on air: pH 7.19, PCO_2 3.7, PO_2 11.5, Bicarbonate 13, Base excess −14

Urinanalysis Red cells 2+

ECG ST elevation in I, II, III, aVF and V_{1-6}

Chest X-ray No pulmonary oedema and heart not obviously enlarged

The most appropriate treatment for this patient is:

A calcium gluconate
B furosemide (frusemide) infusion
C haemodialysis
D pericardiocentesis
E thrombolysis

Answers

2.1   **C***** A non-insulin dependent diabetic (NIDDM) suffers an anterior MI and now has to be put back onto diabetic medication. According to the DIGAMI study, diabetics who suffer MI have a higher mortality. Patients given intensive intravenous insulin in the acute phase and then put on to 3 months of subcutaneous insulin had an absolute reduction in mortality of 11% at 3.5 years compared to patients left on oral hypoglycaemics.

Malmberg K. (1997) Prospective randomised study of intensive insulin treatment on long term survival after acute myocardial infarction in patients with diabetes mellitus. DIGAMI (Diabetes Mellitus, Insulin Glucose Infusion in Acute Myocardial Infarction) Study Group. *BMJ* **314(7093)**:1512–15.

2.2   **B***** The ECG trace shows ventricular fibrillation and this patient is in cardiac arrest. The most important step in his management is to defibrillate as soon as possible, with the aim of giving three shocks within the first 45 seconds.

2.3   **A***** She has most likely taken a tricyclic antidepressant overdose, as the signs are those of anticholinergic effects, including sinus tachycardia, pyrexia, dry mouth and tongue, dilated pupils and urinary retention. In severe cases, there may be increased tone and hyperreflexia with extensor plantars.

2.4   **A**** This patient has cutaneous larva migrans, caused by migration of nematode larva through intact skin epidermis. The larvae, which originate from dog faeces, live in damp earth or beaches. The migration shows a characteristic zigzag line. *Borrelia burgdorferi* causes Lyme disease. *Trichophyton mentagrophytes* causes ringworm. *Treponema pertenue* causes yaws, a non-venereal infectious condition similar to syphilis. *Ascaris lumbricoides* causes urticaria, eosinophilia and diarrhoea and transient eosinophilic infiltrates (Löfflers syndrome).

2.5   **E***** An elderly woman presents in a drowsy condition with possible urinary tract infection complicated by high glucose, high sodium and minimal acidosis and ketosis. The clinical presentation may mimic DKA except that there are few or no ketones in the urine unless the patient has been starving or vomiting. The plasma glucose is very high; it is rare for insulin dependent diabetics (the type who develop DKA) to present with such a high plasma glucose. The plasma osmolality can be calculated from the following formula:

Serum osmolality = 2 × ([Na] + [K]) + [urea] + [glucose]

In the present case this would be 373 mosmol/kg. Diabetes insipidus is associated with high serum sodium and high serum osmolality but also a low urinary osmolality, which is not the case here. Cushing's syndrome can present with hyperglycaemia and weakness but there are none of the classical features to suggest this as a viable diagnosis.

2.6 **D**** A cross-sectional study would involve surveying all patients with hepatic encephalopathy at a particular point in time to see if they had raised ammonia, and so generate a possible association between the two. This type of study can be used to assess the prevalence of a disease.

2.7 **B**** The diagnosis is intra-abdominal lymphoma causing obstruction at the porta hepatis. It could also be cholangiocarcinoma. If sclerosing cholangitis were the diagnosis then ERCP would be the investigation that would establish the diagnosis. Percutaneous transhepatic cholangiography is used to cannulate the common bile duct if ERCP is not possible. In this case, CT abdomen with biopsy of an intra-abdominal mass would be the investigation of choice.

2.8 **E**** This patient presents with lethargy, weight loss, loss of vision and splenomegaly. The blood results show macrocytic anaemia, lymphocytosis, very raised ESR and raised IgM. Although there is evidence of immuno-paresis, the skeletal survey is normal and IgM myeloma is unusual. More likely would be Waldenstrom's macroglobulinaemia, which is usually associated with a raised Ig M gammopathy. As with myeloma, Waldenstrom's macro-globulinaemia causes a hyperviscosity syndrome that can result in headaches, cerebrovascular accidents, and thromboses. The photo shows central retinal vein thrombosis.

2.9 **B*** HIV attacks CD4 cells and causes problems with cell-mediated immunity. As a result such patients are at risk of opportunistic infections by viruses, fungi and mycobacterium. By contrast *Haemophilus influenzae* is an encapsu-lated bacterium and poses more of a threat to patients who lack humoral immunity (i.e. splenectomy patients), as they are unable to produce opsoniz-ing antibodies.

2.10 **A**** The histology slide shows large bowel and in the centre of the picture is a granuloma with surrounding inflammation. This is characteristic of Crohn's disease, as ulcerative colitis is not associated with granulomas.

2.11 **A***** Pyrexia, tender hepatomegaly without jaundice and normal liver function tests are characteristic of an amoebic liver abscess. The most likely organism would be *Entamoeba histolytica*, which is a protozoan with a world-wide distribution. This could be a bacterial pyogenic hepatic abscess but patients tend to be older, much more unwell and more associated with enteric symptoms. Hydatid cysts are associated with a much longer history of abdominal distension in patients who rear sheep or cattle. The normal eosinophil count makes schistosomiasis unlikely and there is no history of haematuria. Hepatitis A would be associated with more deranged liver function tests and jaundice.

2.12 A** This patient is most likely to have had a cerebral infarct due to embolism, given his history of atrial fibrillation. There is evidence that he should be started on aspirin 300 mg as an antiplatelet drug. Intracranial thrombolysis is a possible treatment if given within 3 hours of the cerebrovascular accident occurring, and in the setting of a neurosurgical centre, and there is exclusion of haemorrhage by CT scan. Warfarin is not indicated in the acute setting.

CAST (Chinese Acute Stroke Trial) Collaborative Group (1997) Randomised placebo-controlled trial of early aspirin use in 20,000 patients with acute ischaemic stroke. *Lancet* **349:**1641–49.

2.13 D*** This patient is diabetic and has multiple discrete circumscribed laser scars in the peripheries and just within the arcades, but sparing the macular region. The patient has had panretinal photocoagulation for proliferative diabetic retinopathy.

2.14 E** This patient has respiratory acidosis, as shown by a low pH and raised PCO_2. The bicarbonate is appropriately raised, suggesting chronic renal adaptation. The PO_2 is low and shows him to have type II respiratory failure. For an explanation of arterial blood gas interpretation, see **1.30.**

2.15 B** Fibromyalgia is a non-inflammatory diffuse pain syndrome of unknown aetiology. Patients may complain of morning stiffness, fatigue, depression, headache, arthralgia and anxiety. Patients may also have other pain syndromes, like irritable bowel syndrome and migraine. On examination there may be certain muscle tender areas like the occiput, supraspinatus and trapezius. Blood results are normal. With polymyalgia rheumatica one would expect an elevated ESR.

2.16 A* Only Behçet's syndrome is not associated with blue sclera. The other four conditions are heritable disorders of type I collagen, which is necessary for the strength of bone, ligaments, tendons and skin.

2.17 C** There is 'egg-shell' calcification of the hilar lymph glands and the most likely diagnosis is sarcoidosis. Differential diagnoses for this appearance include silicosis and pneumoconiosis. Hodgkin's lymphoma can produce bihilar lymphadenopathy but not calcification.

2.18 E** This plain abdominal X-ray reveals fusion of the vertebral bodies and calcification of the longitudinal ligaments and intervertebral discs consistent with ankylosing spondylitis. Ankylosing spondylitis is associated with iritis, not scleritis.

2.19 D** With cardiac catheterisation the oxygen saturation on the right side of the heart should be 65–75%, whereas the saturation on the left side of the heart should be 96–98%. All the oxygen saturations on the right side should be the same: superior vena cava, inferior vena cava, right atrium, right ventricle and pulmonary artery; the oxygen saturations on the left should also be the same, only more oxygenated. The first chamber to show a deviation of greater than >5% in the oxygen saturation is where the shunt is. In this case there is an increase in the oxygen saturation from the right ventricle to the pulmonary artery consistent with a patent ductus arteriosus. The elevated pulmonary artery pressure suggests that the patient has developed pulmonary hypertension.

2.20 A** On the pre-treatment ECG (A), there are peaked T waves in V_{1-6} and a broad QRS complex and prolonged PR interval, which would be consistent with hyperkalaemia. The treatment of choice would be 10ml 10% calcium gluconate to protect the myocardium, followed by insulin-dextrose infusion to reduce the hyperkalaemia. The post-treatment ECG (B) shows the reduction in size of the T waves after treatment.

2.21 C** This patient presents with the characteristic features of lithium toxicity: vomiting, incontinence, tremor, myoclonic jerks and restlessness. Other features include hypernatraemia, convulsions, arrhythmias, cerebellar signs and renal failure. There is no specific antidote for lithium overdose but if there are neurological sequelae then haemodialysis should be considered.

2.22 D** Porphyria cutanea tarda is a disorder of porphyrin biosynthesis where there is a deficiency of uroporphyrinogen III decarboxylase in the liver; as a result there is increased production of urinary uroporphyrin. In porphyria cutanea tarda there are no neurological sequelae but it is associated with chronic liver damage. Patients develop characteristic skin lesions: photo-sensitive skin blisters that heal with scarring; increased skin fragility; hyper-trichosis and alopecia; and rarely a 'pseudoscleroderma' where there is extensive sclerosis and thickening of the skin. Epidermolysis bullosa involves blistering of the skin occurring in parts of the body exposed to trauma or friction, like hands and soles of feet.

2.23 D* This patient has suffered a myocardial infarction. Her thyroid function tests show a slightly low TSH and a slightly low free T_4. Given the fact that she has undergone a major physical stress it is very difficult to interpret her true thyroid status. The thyroid function tests should return back to normal after she recovers.

2.24 D* Odds ratio is a measure of risk calculated by comparing the odds or probability an event will occur in an experimental group compared within a control group. The closer the value is to 1, the smaller is the difference in effect between the two groups' exposure to the risk factor. When events are rare, OR is analogous to RR.

	Leukaemia +	Leukaemia −	
Exposure to power cables	10 (a)	30 (b)	40
Non-exposure to power cables	40 (c)	80 (d)	120
	50	110	160

Odds for developing leukaemia = number exposed to risk factor/number not exposed = 10/40 = a/c

Odds for controls = number exposed to risk factor/number not exposed = 30/80 = b/d

OR = (a/c)/(b/d) = (ad)/(bc) = $(10 \times 80)/(30 \times 40)$ = 0.67

2.25 A, E, I** A patient with decompensated liver disease, presumably due to alcoholic liver disease, presents with mild ascites, jaundice and early encephalopathy. He is homeless and so is likely to have poor nutrition, and hence thiamine deficiency is a distinct possibility. Intravenous thiamine (Pabrinex) is a very effective method of correcting any deficiency and certainly this should be started before giving dextrose, as dextrose may precipitate encephalopathy. Oral lactulose to prevent constipation and so reduce the bowel flora may be the single most useful drug given to any patient with decompensated liver disease to prevent encephalopathy. Spontaneous bacterial peritonitis must be excluded in any patient with ascites and fluid should be sent for culture and white cell count; a value of 250 cells/cm^3 is diagnostic of spontaneous bacterial peritonitis and antibiotics should then be started.

2.26 E** This patient has von Willebrand's disease, which is an abnormality of the factor VIII von Willebrand's factor and is usually inherited in an autosomal dominant manner. The disease is characterised by an increased bleeding time and reduced levels of factor VIII coagulant activity. Here there is no circulating antibody to factor VIII because there is a reduction of the APTT on mixing the plasma with normal plasma. He has a normal factor IX level, thereby excluding haemophilia B.

2.27 A* The slide shows surface villi with goblet cells, which stain light blue with mucin. As this shows intestinal metaplasia of the normal squamous epithelium, this is Barrett's oesophagus (see **5.15**). Carcinoma would show invasion. Candida is not seen in glandular epithelium; it would be found with squamous epithelial cells showing the hyphae.

2.28 D** A patient with fever, haematuria, dry cough and eosinophilia should suggest a worm infestation. None of the other options is associated with eosinophilia (>0.4). The most likely organism is *Schistosoma haematobium* contracted while swimming. Patients may also complain of pruritus and urticaria, diarrhoea and have patchy pneumonia on chest X-ray. Diagnosis involves microscopy of terminal urine and treatment is with mebendazole.

2.29 A** He has a motor and sensory neuropathy with pes cavus and absent plantar reflexes. The gait is due to bilateral foot drop and so patients appear to drag their feet. This is Charcot-Marie-Tooth disease or hereditary motor and sensory neuropathy (HSMN) and it is a form of peripheral neuropathy. Classically patients are said to have 'inverted champagne bottles' to describe the pattern of muscle wasting in the legs and thickened lateral popliteal and great auricular nerves. There may be a family history.

2.30 E*** This patient has respiratory alkalosis, as shown by a raised pH and low PCO_2. Her bicarbonate and base excess are normal so there is no evidence of metabolic alkalosis. The PO_2 is normal so there is no respiratory failure. These results would be consistent with hyperventilation. For an explanation of arterial blood gas interpretation, see **1.30**.

2.31 E*** This man presents with oedema secondary to nephrotic syndrome, congestive cardiac failure, hepatomegaly, carpal tunnel syndrome and macro-glossia. The most likely diagnosis is amyloidosis, which is a condition whereby proteinaceous material is deposited in the extracellular matrix of tissues. Amyloidosis may be primary/idiopathic, associated with myeloma, be associated with renal dialysis or secondary to infections like tuberculosis, neoplasms like lymphoma and other chronic conditions like rheumatoid arthritis. HOCM, constrictive pericarditis and carcinoid could explain the heart failure and hepatomegaly but not the macroglossia and nephrotic syndrome.

2.32 A* The photograph shows large separation between the individual teeth characteristic of acromegaly. Amyloidosis, vitamin B_{12} deficiency and hypo-thyroidism affect the tongue. Vitamin C deficiency causes bleeding and ulcerated gums.

2.33 D** This patient is most likely to complain of odynophagia (pain on swallow-ing), as her predominant symptom. There are multiple small filling defects in long columns. Contrast this image with the one of oesophageal varices (see **5.32**).

2.34 A* This patient has a history and blood results suggestive of encephalitis. Encephalitis may follow a viral prodrome but can present acutely as well. The MRI shows involvement of the left temporal lobe, accounting for her memory problems. The treatment is high dose aciclovir.

2.35 B** This patient presents with low grade fever and pleuritic chest dis-comfort and has an extra heart sound, which could be a pericardial rub. The diagnosis is Dressler's syndrome, which is an acute pericarditis of unknown aetiology that may complicate myocardial infarction. It tends to present 10 days to 2 months postinfarct. Patients may also present with pleural and pericardial effusions and arthralgia. The most effective treatment is anti-inflammatory drugs.

2.36 **B**** The ECG shows a regular broad complex tachycardia with right bundle branch block. He has no history of ischaemic heart disease and is haemo-dynamically stable. There are none of the features of ventricular tachycardia (see **3.35**).

2.37 **F, I, J*** This patient has pyoderma gangrenosum, which is a chronic ulcer that has a necrotic ulcer base and dark red or violaceous border. It is associated with all the conditions mentioned, including other malignancies, endocrinopathies like diabetes mellitus and hypothyroidism, and liver diseases like primary biliary cirrhosis.

2.38 **D*** This patient with hypocalcaemia has pseudohypoparathyroidism. In this condition patients have raised PTH because it is ineffective at the target organ. Vitamin D_3 is converted to 25-vitamin D_3 in the liver and then to 1,25-vitamin D_3 in the kidney. In cirrhosis there are decreased levels of 25-vitamin D_3 and also albumin, which is produced by the liver. Patients with pseudo-hypoparathyroidism have a short stature, short fourth and fifth metacarpals and mental retardation. Pseudopseudohypoparathyroidism has the clinical features of pseudohypoparathyroidism but the serum calcium and other bio-chemical values are normal.

2.39 **B*** Jehovah's Witnesses are forbidden to have certain transfusions and these include red cells, white cells, platelets and plasma. They cannot receive their own blood even if they donated it prior to an operation. However, they can receive their own blood if it is transfused back into them during an operation, provided that the blood has been through a salvage machine or cell saver whereby the red cells have been separated and 'washed out'. Other blood products that are acceptable include albumin, clotting factors like factors VIII and IX, erythropoietin and immunoglobulins.

2.40 **B**** Coeliac disease is a malabsorption syndrome associated with sensitivity to gluten. Patients may have a moderate macrocytic anaemia due to folate deficiency, and microcytosis due to iron malabsorption. Duodenal or jejunal biopsies typically show villous atrophy with crypt hyperplasia; crypt abscesses are a characteristic of ulcerative colitis. Antiendomyseal, antigliadin and tissue transglutaminase antibodies are IgA and so may be normal in a coeliac patient who has IgA – deficiency in that case IgA antigliadin should be checked.

2.41 **E**** This patient has Wolff–Parkinson–White syndrome, which is a form of atrioventricular re-entry tachycardia. WPW is caused by an accessory AV pathway (bundle of Kent), which connects atrial and ventricular myocardium and bypasses the AV node and bundle of His. Patients with WPW may develop paroxysmal tachycardias and atrial fibrillation. Drugs like verapamil and digoxin block the AV node and can increase the frequency of conduction in the accessory pathway, so leading to faster ventricular rate. The other drugs slow conduction in the accessory pathway.

2.42 A** The likely diagnosis is Goodpasture's syndrome. This is a type II hypersensitivity condition characterised by circulating anti-GBM antibodies and linear deposition of immunoglobulin and complement in the GBM, resulting in pulmonary haemorrhage and renal failure. Additional aetiological factors are that he is a young male smoker presenting with severe acute renal failure. A less likely diagnosis is Wegener's granulomatosis but this is characterised by positive c-ANCA.

2.43 E** This patient presents with chronic sinusitis, lower respiratory tract inflammation, renal impairment, sensory neuropathy, vasculitic skin lesion and characteristic chest X-ray signs. The serum ANCA is not given but the most likely diagnosis is Wegener's granulmatosis. SLE is unlikely as she is ANA-negative and has normal serum complement, also making it unlikely to be mixed cryoglobulinaemia. Goodpasture's syndrome is characterised by pulmonary haemorrhage and glomerulonephritis but cannot explain the other findings.

2.44 E*** In Paget's disease there is uncontrolled bone metabolism. There is bone resorption due to osteoclast activity and in the skull this can produce a honeycomb appearance, 'osteoporosis circumscripta'. There is bone demineralisation resulting in a sharp contrast occurring between normal and abnormal bone. There is also increased osteoblastic activity which can give a cotton wool appearance. Other deformities that may occur include basilar invagination and platybasia. Myeloma and metastases would show a skull with punched-out lesions, not bone sclerosis (except with some prostate cancers).

2.45 D*** This patient has soft tissue loss of the terminal phalanges of the right index and middle fingers. This type of destruction is characteristic of systemic sclerosis.

2.46 A** This patient has a myopathy with wasting of facial, shoulder and girdle muscles. The reflexes are absent because of muscle atrophy. The ptosis and slurred speech are all consistent with dystrophia myotonia. Other features include percussion dystonia, inability to relax a clenched fist and frontal baldness. The diabetes is due to end-organ unresponsiveness to insulin. Compare this with 4.11.

2.47 E* A severely malnourished person is suddenly given large amounts of kilocalories in the form of intravenous dextrose and nasogastric feed. This has caused salt and volume overload, resulting in low levels of potassium, phosphorus and magnesium. The way to avoid this is to give less than his calculated nutritional requirements and slowly build up his energy intake. Simple fluid overload is unlikely to cause electrolyte imbalances. Kwashiorkor is a form of protein-calorie malnutrition characterised by fatigue, irritability, decreased immunity, loss of muscle bulk and generalized oedema.

2.48 B* This patient has Parkinson's syndrome. The treatment that should not be given to this patient would be a dopamine depleter like tetrabenazine or reserpine. Baclofen can be used to treat dystonia, especially caused by levodopa. Entacapone is a catechol-*o*-methyl transferase inhibitor which prevents the degradation of dopamine. Apomorphine and bromocriptine are dopamine agonists.

2.49 A** Long-term oxygen therapy has been shown to improve the mortality rate in patients with COPD if they have continuous delivery of oxygen via nasal prongs or mask for at least 15 hours per day. The oxygen concentration is 1–3 Litres/min given via a FiO_2 28% mask. However the benefits have only been shown in patients who have a FEV_1 ≤1.5 Litres and who have a PO_2 ≤7.3 kPa (or 8.0 kPa if there is evidence of pulmonary hypertension). The oxygen status needs to be assessed at least 30 days after recovery from an acute exacerbation of COPD and must be done on room air. Patients must not smoke in case they ignite themselves but exercise tolerance does not determine whether or not patients should receive long-term oxygen therapy.

Medical Research Council Working Party (1981) Long-term domicillary oxygen therapy in chronic hypoxic cor pulmonale complicating chronic bronchitis and emphysema. *Lancet* 1:681–86.

2.50 D* The most likely diagnosis is steroid-induced osteonecrosis or avascular necrosis of the femoral head. Her DEXA scan is normal (for DEXA scan interpretation, see **1.7**), and she has no biochemical evidence of osteomalacia. It would be unusual to have purely osteoarthritis affecting one hip without a history of trauma. Collapse of the articular surface is characteristic of osteonecrosis.

2.51 C** There are multiple foci with increased signal in the periventricular white matter. This would be consistent with multiple sclerosis. A differential diagnosis would be multiple cerebral infarcts. The ventricles are not increased in size. A definitive diagnosis of multiple sclerosis would require looking for oligoclonal bands in the CSF.

2.52 E** This patient has a black-pigmented nodule that has an irregular margin, which looks like a malignant melanoma. Poor prognostic features include: lesion diameter ≥2.0 cm; Breslow lesion thickness ≥7.5 mm; lesions involving mucosae, anorectal and vulval regions because such areas are not routinely checked and so lesions have become deeply penetrated at the time of diagnosis; amelanotic malignant melanomas are more difficult to diagnose and are also more aggressive tumours. Males tend to present with tumours on their face and back rather than females, who tend to develop them on the sun-exposed parts of their legs.

2.53 B* This girl presents with primary amenorrhoea. She has normal breast development and normal female external genitalia but male internal genitalia. She is genotypically a male but phenotypically a female. This is complete androgen insensitivity. Breasts develop normally because excess testosterone secretion is converted to oestrogen. Development of male external genitalia depends on normal testosterone synthesis, conversion to dihydrotestosterone and normal androgen receptors. Because of her karyotype the patient produces Müllerian inhibitory factor; there is no uterus, cervix or ovaries. With gonadal dysgenesis there is maldevelopment of the testes. As there is the risk of malignancy with intra-abdominal or maldeveloped testes, orchidopexy should be performed. Klinefelter's syndrome patients would usually have a karyotype of 47,XXY. She does not have the phenotypic features of Kallman's syndrome (see **1.55**). The normal 17-OH progesterone excludes 11-β-hydroxylase deficiency.

2.54 B** This patient has Dukes' C_2 carcinoma of the colon. For a description of the grading system, see Question 1.14. The 5-year survival rate with treatment depends on the Dukes' grading of the tumour: A is 95–100%; B_1 is 85%; B_2 is 75%; C_1 is 65%; C_2 is 40%; and D is 5–10%.

2.55 B* This patient has Turner's syndrome, which is associated with karyotype 45,XO but many patients have a mosaic form such as 46,XX/45,XO especially if they do not display many of the distinctive features such as cubitus valgus (wide carrying angle), epicanthic folds, low set ears, neck webbing and shield-like chest with widely spaced nipples. Only 20% of patients have cardiac abnormalities like coarctation of the aorta; over 60% have renal anomalies. Patients will require oestrogen sex hormone replacement but, unopposed, this can lead to endometrial hyperplasia and possibly carcinoma; progesterone will also have to be prescribed with cyclical oestrogen to ensure a withdrawal bleed. Growth hormone may improve longitudinal growth and final height.

2.56 A** This patient has all the hallmarks of cholangitis. Even though the gallbladder has been removed, there is still the possibility that gallstones may occur in the common bile duct.

2.57 A** This patient has a gastrinoma. The watery diarrhoea along with the excessive gastin production is associated with the Zollinger–Ellison syndrome. Normally, secretin infusion should cause a decrease in gastrin secretion but with gastrinomas there is a paradoxical increase. Verner–Morrison syndrome is due to a tumour secreting VIP and is associated with watery diarrhoea, hypokalaemia and achlorhydria (WDHA syndrome). All of these tumours can arise from the pancreas.

2.58 **C***** This patient has developed pyridoxine (vitamin B$_6$) deficiency due to her isoniazid treatment. It might possibly have been avoided if she had been coprescribed this at the start of her antituberculosis treatment.

2.59 **C**** The echocardiogram shows a thick interventricular septum and dilated left ventricle consistent with HOCM.

2.60 **C**** An elderly woman develops acute renal failure in the postoperative period after being treated with non-steroidal anti-inflammatory drugs (NSAIDs) and antibiotics. She has clinical evidence of pericarditis, as shown by ECG changes and extra heart sounds. She has a number of indications for haemodialysis: raised potassium, metabolic acidosis and uraemic pericarditis. Other indications for haemodialysis include resistant fluid overload, multi-organ failure, hypercalcaemia, hypercatabolic states and drug toxicities. An echocardiogram would need to be done to exclude a pericardial effusion but unless the patient clinically had tamponade, pericardiocentesis should not be attempted.

Paper 3

Questions

3.1 A 63-year-old woman suffered a myocardial infarction. She was treated by thrombolysis and made a good recovery so that 3 days later she was completely pain free and mobilising. She had no previous medical problems.

On examination she was apyrexial, pulse 80 regular and blood pressure 125/78. Cardiovascular and respiratory examinations were normal.

The most important contraindication to exercise testing would be if the patient:

A develops a febrile illness
B has a permanent pacemaker
C is on atenolol
D exhibits LBBB on a resting ECG
E was six days post infarct

3.2 A 74-year-old woman collapsed at home and was brought to the Accident & Emergency department.

Her ECG shows:

A 1st degree AV block
B complete heart block
C Mobitz type I 2nd degree AV block
D Mobitz type II 2nd degree AV block
E sinus bradycardia

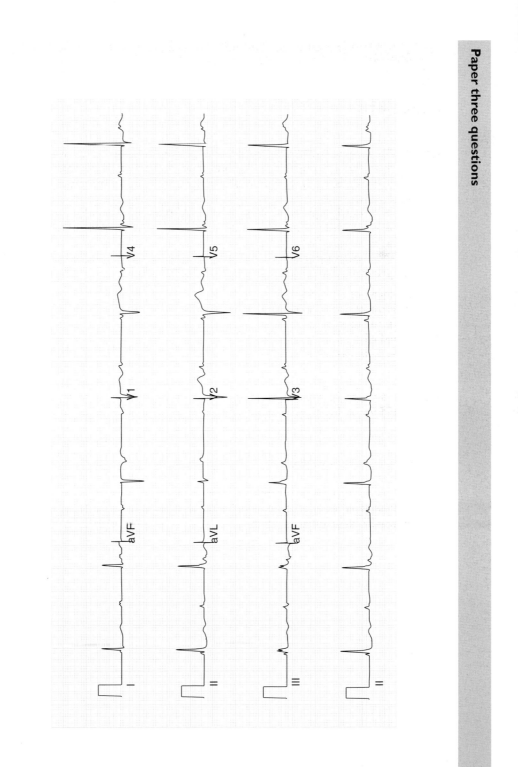

3.3 A 52-year-old farmer was admitted to Accident & Emergency with an overdose of an insecticide taken 18 hours ago. He complained of lethargy, dizziness, headache, vomiting and abdominal pain followed by shortness of breath and non-productive cough. Now he could not speak in full sentences.

On examination he was alert but breathless. His temperature was 36.9°C, pulse 55 regular and blood pressure 110/65. His JVP was not elevated and heart sounds were normal. His respiratory rate was 26 breaths/min and there was bilateral wheeze. He had generalised abdominal tenderness.

Arterial blood	pH	7.45	PCO_2	3.4
gases on air	PO_2	9.9	Bicarbonate	20.9
	Base excess	−3.1		

The correct antidote for this patient is:

    A atropine
    B sodium bicarbonate
    C dimercaprol
    D glucagon
    E procyclidine

3.4 A 35-year-old farmer presented with a tender itchy lesion on his right index finger that developed 5 days ago after feeding lambs. He had no other symptoms (Figure 3.4). See plate section.

The most likely diagnosis is:

    A Anthrax
    B Herpetic whitlow
    C *Molluscum contagiosum*
    D Orf
    E Tinea manum

3.5 A 65-year-old man presented with headaches and worsening lower limb pain, making walking difficult. He felt that his problems had been worse over the last several months. He had smoked 20 cigarettes a day for nearly 50 years. His appetite was normal but he had lost some weight.

On examination he was apyrexial. Cardiovascular and respiratory examination were normal. There was no focal neurological deficit.

Bloods	Hb	14.2	WCC	8.5
	Platelets	246	Na	142
	K	3.9	Urea	7.8
	Creatinine	80	Calcium	2.30
	Phosphate	1.0	Albumin	39
	ALP	130	Protein	68

Pelvic X-ray Figure 3.5. See plate section.

The most likely diagnosis is:

A multiple myeloma
B osteomalacia
C Paget's disease
D primary hyperparathyroidism
E secondary metastases from lung carcinoma

3.6 It had been reported that living close to mobile phone masts was associated with an increased risk of developing brain tumours. You have been asked to design a study to investigate this possibility.

The most appropriate study design would be:

A case control study
B case reports
C cohort study
D cross-sectional study
E randomised control trial

3.7 A 28-year-old man presented with a history of dark urine and pale stools for the past 3 weeks. Prior to this he had developed intractable itching, which did not respond to chlorphenamine (chlorpheniramine). For the past 5 years he had also suffered from loose stools with occasional blood in the motions. He had no other medical problems. He had not travelled abroad and he did not drink or smoke.

On examination he was very jaundiced but was well built. There was no lymphadenopathy but he had a palpable liver edge.

Bloods				
	Hb	11.4	WCC	11.1
	Platelets	172	INR	1.0
	Na	140	K	3.8
	Urea	3.6	Creatinine	95
	Bilirubin	108	Albumin	36
	Protein	64	ALP	500
	AST	60	GGT	40
	ESR	18	CRP	20

Hepatitis A, B, C serology Negative

Stool culture Negative

Abdominal ultrasound
Hepatomegaly; no splenomegaly
Normal common bile duct; gallbladder empty
Dilated intrahepatic ducts

Sigmoidoscopy Mildly inflamed mucosa

The most helpful test to establish the diagnosis is:

A antimitochondrial antibodies
B CT abdomen
C ERCP
D MRCP
E ultrasound-guided liver biopsy

3.8 A 13-year-old boy was referred with recurrent attacks of abdominal pain and jaundice. This was the fourth time it had happened but previously these attacks had resolved spontaneously. Three days ago he had developed a sore throat, myalgia and headache. He had no previous medical history and was not on any medication.

On examination he was mildly jaundiced. His temperature was 37.3°C, pulse 98 regular and blood pressure 100/65. Cardiovascular and respiratory examination were normal. On palpation of his abdomen he had 4 cm splenomegaly.

Bloods	Hb	11.5	MCV	100.1
	WCC	3.9	Platelets	150
	Protein	70	Albumin	40
	Bilirubin	43	ALT	25
	ALP	600	GGT	35

Urinanalysis Urobilinogen 2+, no bilirubin

Direct Coombs' test Negative

The most helpful test to determine the definitive diagnosis would be:

 A bone marrow aspirate and trephine
 B haemoglobin electrophoresis
 C Ham's test
 D osmotic fragility studies
 E Schumm's test

3.9 A 46-year-old man was referred with abdominal pain and chronic diarrhoea. He opened his bowels 3–4 times per day and his stools were loose and occasionally associated with mucus. His symptoms started 5 months ago after he had returned from working in Sri Lanka for the past 3 years. His appetite was decreased and he had lost some weight. He had no other medical problems and was not on any medication. He did not smoke or drink alcohol.

On examination he was apyrexial, pulse 78 regular and blood pressure 134/79. Abdominal examination revealed general tenderness. Rectal examination was normal. A duodenal (D2) biopsy was taken at endoscopy (Figure 3.9). See plate section.

The most likely diagnosis is:

 A coeliac disease
 B Crohn's disease
 C giardiasis
 D tropical sprue
 E Whipple's disease

3.10 A 24-year-old man presented with epistaxis, haematemesis and melaena for one day. Since arriving back in the UK from Burma 5 days ago he had been having a flu-like illness associated with abdominal pain. He had taken malaria prophylaxis before he went. He had no significant previous medical history and was not on any medication except mefloquine.

On examination he looked unwell and jaundiced. There were non-blanching erythematous bruises on his skin. His temperature was 39°C, pulse 110 regular and blood pressure 96/64. Respiratory examination was normal. He had diffuse abdominal tenderness but no organo-megaly or lymphadenopathy. Rectal examination revealed melaena.

Bloods				
Hb	11.1	WCC	2.8
Neutrophils	1.4	Lymphocytes	1.1
Eosinophils	0.1	Monocytes	0.2
Platelets	90	Na	130
K	5.0	Urea	12.1
Creatinine	200	Protein	58
Albumin	28	Bilirubin	75
ALT	80	ALP	130

Malaria films Negative

Urinanalysis Protein 3+, blood 3+

Chest X-ray Normal

The most likely diagnosis is:

   A blackwater fever
   B dengue haemorrhagic fever
   C hepatitis A
   D typhoid
   E yellow fever

3.11 A 50-year-old man presented with progressive weakness. He had difficulty walking and climbing upstairs and more recently combing his hair. Over the last few months he noticed decreased appetite, some weight loss and some dysphagia for solids. There was no previous medical history. He did not smoke or drink alcohol.

On examination he had bilateral wasting of both shoulders and quadriceps. There were no ocular or facial abnormalities. He had normal tone, power and reflexes. Apart from atrial fibrillation with a rate of 88 there was no other abnormality to be found on examination.

The most likely diagnosis is:

A limb–girdle muscular dystrophy
B myasthenia gravis
C motor neurone disease
D polymyalgia rheumatica
E polymyositis

3.12 A 38-year-old diabetic man was referred to the eye clinic by the optician. Fundoscopy was performed and is shown below (Figure 3.12). See plate section.

The fundoscopic appearance is most likely to be due to:

A choroidal melanoma
B diabetic maculopathy
C preretinal haemorrhage
D retinal detachment
E toxoplasma scar

3.13 A patient was referred for lung function tests:

	Absolute	Predicted (%)
FEV_1	1.8	51
FVC	2.4	55
TLC	3.0	52
DLCO	12.0	53
KCO	5.0	99

These results could be consistent with which **TWO** of the following:

A asthma
B bronchiectasis
C chronic bronchitis
D emphysema
E fibrosing alveolitis
F lymphangitis carcinomatosa
G patient post pneumonectomy for lung carcinoma
H primary pulmonary hypertension
I pulmonary haemorrhage
J sarcoidosis

3.14 A 51-year-old woman was referred because of worsening joint pain affecting her hands. The problems started about 4 months ago causing pain in both wrists and now the fingers were involved. She was unable to perform her job as a typist. Simple analgesics had not helped her symptoms. She had no previous medical history and was only on codeine phosphate.

On examination she was in pain. She had bilateral swelling and tenderness affecting wrists, metacarpophalangeal joints and proximal interphalangeal joints. Sensation was normal. She was unable to oppose her fingers.

Which **ONE** of the following is associated with a **BETTER** prognosis for her condition?

    A Acute onset
    B Early erosions on imaging
    C Presence of HLA-DR4 genetic marker
    D Presence of subcutaneous nodules
    E Rheumatoid factor seropositivity

3.15 This 65-year-old man presented with a long history of progressive weakness (Figure 3.15). See plate section.

The most likely diagnosis is:

    A Becker's muscular dystrophy
    B dystrophia myotonica
    C hypothyroidism
    D myasthenia gravis
    E Parkinson's syndrome

3.16 A 64-year-old man was referred because of alternating constipation and diarrhoea over the past 4 weeks (Figure 3.16). See plate section.

The most significant abnormality on the barium enema is:

    A colonic carcinoma
    B Crohn's colitis
    C diverticular disease
    D ischaemic colitis
    E ulcerative colitis

3.17 A 59-year-old man was referred because of progressive jaundice and weight loss. An ERCP was performed (Figure 3.17). See plate section.

The most likely diagnosis is:

A carcinoma of the head of the pancreas
B gallstones obstructing the common bile duct
C normal ERCP
D primary biliary cirrhosis
E primary sclerosing cholangitis

3.18 A 12-year-old boy was referred for cardiac catheterisation because of progressive shortness of breath.

	Pressure	Normal value	O_2 saturation
	(systolic/diastolic, mmHg)		(%)
Right atrium (mean)	8	0–8	75
Right ventricle	28/8	15–30/0–8	84
Pulmonary artery	45/15	15–30/0–8	85
Left atrium (mean)	12	1–10	96
Left ventricle	132/12	100–140/3–12	97
Aorta	135/70	100–140/60–90	97

The most likely diagnosis is:

A atrial septal defect
B coarctation of the aorta
C Fallot's tetralogy
D patent ductus arteriosus
E ventricular septal defect

3.19 A 56-year-old man was admitted with an inferior MI for which he was treated with thrombolysis. Three hours later he became cold, clammy and short of breath. He continued to have a pulse.

The ECG shows:

    A supraventricular tachycardia with aberrant conduction
    B atrial fibrillation with aberrant conduction
    C torsades de pointes
    D ventricular fibrillation
    E ventricular standstill

3.20 A 59-year-old homeless man was admitted with abdominal pain, vomiting, dizziness and blurred vision. He was a chronic alcoholic and confirmed he had drunk methylated spirits about 5 hours ago. He had no other medical problems and was on no medication.

    On examination his GCS score was 14/15. His temperature was 37.2°C, pulse 86 regular and blood pressure 138/90. His respiratory rate was 26 breaths/min and his chest was clear. There was diffuse abdominal tenderness. He was uncooperative with neurological examination but appeared to have decreased visual acuity.

Arterial blood	pH	7.18	PCO_2	3.4
gases on air	PO_2	10.1	Bicarbonate	12.4
	Base excess	−13.5		

Which **ONE** of the following concerning this patient's management is **FALSE?**

    A Activated charcoal should be given
    B Haemodialysis is indicated if mental or visual features are present
    C Intravenous bicarbonate should be given
    D Ipecacuanha is contraindicated
    E Oral ethanol should be given

3.21 A 25-year-old man was admitted with community-acquired pneumonia. Two days later he developed this non-pruritic skin rash on both legs, both arms and in his mouth (Figure 3.21). See plate section.

The skin lesion is mostly like to be:

    A allergic reaction to penicillin
    B erythema multiforme
    C erythema nodosum
    D guttate psoriasis
    E pyoderma gangrenosum

3.22 A 70-year-old woman was brought to casualty in a confused state. She was found collapsed at home and unable to provide a reliable history. Her old notes documented a history of ischaemic heart disease and treatment with radioiodine. She denied any chest pain but did complain of a non-productive cough. She was taking low dose aspirin and a glyceryl trinitrate spray.

On examination she was pale and had a temperature of 33.4°C. Her pulse was 55 regular and blood pressure 95/40. She had bilateral crackles in both bases of her chest. Abdominal examination revealed some generalised tenderness.

Which of the following would **NOT** be an appropriate treatment step in this patient?

A High dose broad-spectrum antibiotics
B Intravenous hydrocortisone 100 mg 8-hourly
C Lugol's iodine solution
D Rewarming the patient
E T_3

3.23 Four hundred patients who had suffered myocardial infarction were followed up to see if continued smoking post-MI was associated with increased risk of dying at the end of 5 years; 100 patients continued to smoke and of these 10 had died, compared with 20 deaths in patients who had stopped smoking. The relative risk (RR) is:

A $(10 \times 30)/(90 \times 370)$
B $(10 \times 100)/(20 \times 300)$
C $(10 \times 280)/(20 \times 90)$
D $(10 \times 300)/(20 \times 100)$
E $(10 \times 370)/(30 \times 90)$

3.24 A 46-year-old woman was referred with progressive abdominal swelling for the past 2 weeks and increasing lethargy. Following this it was noticed that she looked yellow. She had no other medical problems. She did not smoke, drink alcohol or take any other medication. She had no relevant family history.

On examination she was jaundiced and had scratch marks on her forearms and abdomen. She was apyrexial, pulse 68 regular and blood pressure 110/55. She had 2 cm hepatomegaly and moderate ascites.

Bloods	Hb	13.4		WCC	4.5
	Platelets	110		MCV	85.4
	Na	132		K	4.8
	Urea	3.9		Creatinine	80
	Albumin	28		Protein	70
	ALT	85		Bilirubin	80
	ALP	105		GGT	39
	INR	1.4			

Antinuclear antibodies	1 in 80
Smooth muscle antibodies	1 in 160
Antimitochondrial antibodies	1 in 16
Anti-DS DNA	Negative
Hepatitis A, B, C serology	Negative
Caeruloplasmin	245

Liver ultrasound   Hepatomegaly but no focal liver lesion

Spleen, pancreas, gallbladder and kidneys normal

Moderate ascites

No common bile duct dilatation

The most likely diagnosis is:

A autoimmune hepatitis
B primary biliary cirrhosis
C primary sclerosing cholangitis
D systemic lupus erythematosus
E Wilson's disease

3.25 A 58-year-old man complained of chest tightness and shortness of breath. He had just had an emergency operation for an aortic aneurysm repair and had been transfused 4 units of blood. Apart from hypercholesterolaemia he had no previous medical history and was on no medication, nor was he allergic to any drugs.

On examination he appeared distressed. His temperature was 40.1°C, pulse 110 regular and blood pressure 90/60. His chest was clear with a respiratory rate of 22 breaths/min. The abdomen was generally tender.

ECG   Sinus tachycardia

Chest X-ray Normal

Urinanalysis Haemoglobin 2+, blood 1+

The most likely complication to have occurred is:

    A acute coronary syndrome
    B bowel perforation
    C circulatory overload
    D pulmonary embolus
    E transfusion reaction

3.26 A 56-year-old man was admitted with worsening abdominal pain associated with vomiting that had been going on for the past 10 days. He had decreased appetite and some weight loss. For the past 4 months he had had a change in his bowel habit with increased frequency but had not opened his bowels for a week. He had no previous medical history and was on no medication.

      On examination he had bilateral ankle oedema. His temperature was 37.4°C, pulse 100 regular and blood pressure 130/80. His abdomen was distended and generally tender with no bowel sounds heard.

Abdominal X-ray   Dilated loops of small bowel

A laparotomy was performed and biopsies of the bowel were taken. (The first slide is high power, the second is low power stained with synaptophysin.) (Figure 3.26). See plate section.

The most likely diagnosis is:

    A adenocarcinoma
    B carcinoid tumour
    C coeliac disease
    D Crohn's disease
    E ischaemic bowel

3.27 A 16-year-old boy was admitted with a 2-week history of fever, malaise, headache and night sweats. He had no cough or shortness of breath. He had some abdominal discomfort and back pain but no bowel or urinary symptoms. His appetite was decreased and he had lost some weight. He had no other medical problems and was on no medication. Two months ago he returned from his native Morocco where he had stayed on his uncle's farm.

      On examination he had cervical lymphadenopathy. His temperature was 37.8°C, pulse 98 and blood pressure 95/60. Heart sounds and chest was clear. There was hepatosplenomegaly but no ascites. There was no neurological deficit.

Bloods	Hb	11.4	WCC	3.0
	Neutrophils	1.6	Lymphocytes	1.2
	Eosinophils	0.2	Platelets	150
	INR	1.0	Na	140
	K	4.2	Urea	3.5
	Creatinine	65	Protein	65
	Albumin	35	Bilirubin	10
	ALT	40	ALP	110
	ESR	60	CRP	48

Malaria films Negative

Chest X-ray Normal

The most likely diagnosis is:

    A brucellosis
    B Hodgkin's lymphoma
    C hydatid cyst
    D schistosomiasis
    E strongyloidiasis

3.28 A 40-year-old woman on the psychiatric ward was referred because of increased thirst, dizziness and polyuria. She was on medication for her depressive illness. No abnormality was found on examination. A water deprivation test was performed:

Time after starting (hours)	Plasma osmolality (mosmol/kg)	Urine osmolality (mosmol/kg)
0	285	310
2	292	350
4	296	418
6	302	498
DDAVP 2 µg given intramuscularly		
8	305	580
Plasma$_{ADH}$ post-water deprivation test:	4 (normal: 3–5 pg/mL)	

The most likely diagnosis in this patient is:

    A complete central diabetes insipidus
    B complete nephrogenic diabetes insipidus
    C partial central diabetes insipidus
    D partial nephrogenic diabetes insipidus
    E primary polydipsia

3.29 A 34-year-old woman presented with shortness of breath. She was a non-smoker.

Arterial blood gases on air	pH	7.51	PCO$_2$	3.9
	PO$_2$	8.5	Bicarbonate	24
	Base excess	−1.2	O$_2$ saturation	90%

These results would be most consistent with:

 A acute exacerbation of chronic obstructive airways disease
 B athlete just finishing a half marathon
 C insulin dependent diabetic not taking insulin because feeling unwell
 D pulmonary embolus
 E salicylate overdose 24 hours postingestion

3.30 A 55-year-old woman was referred because of a 1-week history of headache and blurred vision. She had had no fits or photophobia. She had a normal appetite and no weight loss. She had no other medical problems.

On examination she was not in pain. Her pulse was 90 regular and blood pressure 145/88. Her JVP was not elevated and both heart sounds were normal. Respiratory and abdominal examination was normal. She did have some scalp tenderness but there was no cranial nerve abnormality and fundoscopic examination was normal. The rest of the nervous system examination was unremarkable. The most useful investigation to establish the diagnosis would be:

 A carotid Doppler ultrasound
 B CT head
 C lumbar puncture and oligoclonal bands
 D MRI head
 F temporal artery biopsy

3.31 This 32-year-old woman was referred for flexible sigmoidoscopy complaining of alternating constipation for which she took lactulose and senna, and loose stools. Her problems had been going on for 6 months. Her appetite was normal, weight was stable and there was no rectal bleeding. Abdominal and rectal examinations were normal (Figure 3.31). See plate section.

The sigmoidoscopy findings are most consistent with:

 A Crohn's disease
 B familial adenomatous polyposis
 C melanosis coli
 D pseudomembranous colitis
 E ulcerative colitis

3.32 A 76-year-old Vietnamese man presented with recent haemoptysis and weight loss. He had smoked 20 cigarettes per day for over 30 years (Figure 3.32). See plate section.

His chest X-ray findings are most likely to be due to:

A aspergilloma
B bronchiectasis
C bronchogenic carcinoma
D mesothelioma
E tuberculosis

3.33 A 53-year-old man presented with shortness of breath and cough. Five days ago he had been to Belgium and returned back to the UK yesterday. Since arrival his breathing had got worse. He also had been having abdominal pain, muscle pains and loose stools. He had no previous medical history and he did not smoke or drink alcohol. He had not been started on any medication.

On examination he was in distress and using his accessory muscles of respiration. His temperature was 39.0°C, pulse 100 regular and blood pressure 95/58. His respiratory rate was 32 breaths/min and he had bronchial breathing and coarse crackles in the right upper zone of the chest. His abdomen was generally tender.

Bloods	Hb	11.8	WCC	20.2
	Neutrophils	18.2	Platelets	300
	Na	131	K	3.5
	Urea	15.6	Creatinine	220
	Albumin	29	Protein	56
	Bilirubin	34	ALT	79
	ALP	137	Calcium	2.55
	Phosphate	0.9	CRP	332
Arterial blood gases on 10 litres O$_2$	pH	7.19	PCO$_2$	3.8
	PO$_2$	6.9	Bicarbonate	8.9
	Base excess	−16		
Chest X ray:	See Figure 3.33			

Apart from ventilatory support the most appropriate drug medication would be:

A ceftriaxone and clarithromycin
B ciprofloxacin and gentamicin
C clarithromycin and rifampicin
D flucloxacillin and gentamicin
E rifampicin, isoniazid, pyrazinamide and ethambutol

3.34 A 28-year-old woman was admitted with pyrexia and confusion. Two days ago her family had noticed her acting strangely, including an inability to name objects. She did not have a cough or any urinary problems. There was no headache, neck stiffness or photophobia but there was a rash. She had no obvious contact with illness.

On examination she had a temperature of 39.0°C. Her pulse was 110 regular and blood pressure 134/79. Her JVP was not elevated but she had a loud pansystolic murmur at the apex that radiated to the axilla and carotids. There were some bilateral basal crackles in her chest. Abdominal examination was normal. She had an abbreviated mini-mental test score of 3/10. There was also some expressive dysphasia. Cranial nerve examination was normal and she was moving all four limbs. She had flat, red, non-tender, blanching spots on her hands.

Bloods	Hb	13.1	WCC	17.5
	Platelets	376	INR	1.2
	Na	139	K	4.7
	Urea	3.8	Creatinine	78
	Albumin	32	Protein	65
	Bilirubin	12	ALT	25
	ALP	67	Calcium	2.22
	ESR	76	CRP	234

Chest X-ray Enlarged heart

No pulmonary oedema

ECG Voltage criteria for left ventricular hypertrophy

The most helpful test to establish the diagnosis would be:

A electroencephalogram
B herpes simplex serology
C lumbar puncture
D transoesophageal echocardiogram
E vaginal swab

3.35 A 68-year-old woman was admitted with palpitations and collapse. She had a previous medical history of hypertension but was not on any medication. She did not drink alcohol or smoke. Her temperature was 37.4°C and blood pressure 115/74.

The ECG shows:

A atrial fibrillation with aberrant conduction
B supraventricular tachycardia with aberrant conduction
C torsades de pointes
D ventricular fibrillation
E ventricular tachycardia

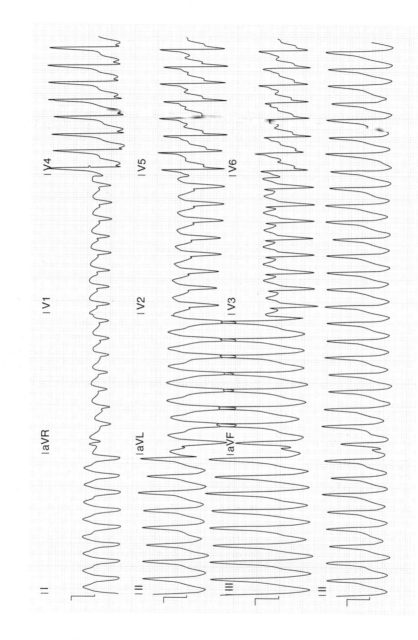

3.36 A 37-year-old woman was referred with a 4-week history of skin changes to both legs (Figure 3.36). See plate section.

The skin rash is:

    A erythema nodosum
    B granuloma annulare
    C lipoatrophy
    D necrobiosis lipoidica
    E tuberous xanthoma

3.37 A 50-year-old man complained of headaches that were getting progressively worse.

CT head   2 cm mass in sella turcica

Which **ONE** of the following complications is **LEAST** likely to occur?

    A Amaurosis fugax
    B Failure to adduct right eye
    C Left complete ptosis and dilated pupil
    D Loss of sensation of lower face and anterior two-thirds of tongue
    E Vertical diplopia on descending stairs

3.38 A 63-year-old man was admitted with a stroke that caused complete expressive dysphasia and right hemiparesis. Initially he was treated with intravenous fluids and then with nasogastric tube feeding. A speech therapist recorded that 2 weeks after developing the stroke he was still at significant risk of aspiration and that PEG feeding would be advisable. The patient, although aphasic, was able to understand commands and was repeatedly warned that his condition would deteriorate if he did not accept feeding. Despite this he kept removing the nasogastric tubes and refused to tolerate further insertions. His family were concerned that the patient appeared to be deteriorating and wanted the PEG tube to be inserted.

    The correct management plan for this patient would be to:

    A ask a psychiatrist to ascertain the mental capability of the patient before deciding
    B insert the PEG tube as requested by the family
    C obtain a court order to insert the PEG tube against the patient's wishes
    D respect the patient's wishes and do not insert the PEG tube or nasogastric tubes
    E wait until the patient becomes unresponsive and then insert the PEG tube

3.39 A 13-year-old boy was brought in with abdominal pain and jaundice. Over the past 2 days he had had diarrhoea and vomiting. Prior to this he had never been ill.

On examination he was apyrexial. He was jaundiced but there was no lymphadenopathy. His pulse was 98 regular and blood pressure 110/70. Respiratory examination was normal. He had mild abdominal tenderness but no organomegaly.

Bloods	Hb	14.0	WCC	5.2
	Platelets	250	INR	1.0
	Bilirubin	60	Albumin	40
	Protein	70	ALT	20
	ALP	500	GGT	20
	Amylase	24		

Urinalysis Urobilinogen 2+, no bilirubin

The most likely diagnosis is:

A biliary atresia
B Dubin–Johnson syndrome
C Gilbert's syndrome
D hereditary spherocytosis
E Rotor syndrome

3.40 A 38-year-old woman presented with a 4-day history of severe pain and paresthesiae in her back radiating down her leg. It came on suddenly and she could not walk. Specifically it affected the buttocks, back and lateral aspects of the thigh and leg and dorsum of the foot. The right side was worse than the left.

On examination she had weakness of her hamstrings, peroneus longus and toe extensors. Tone was normal but power was reduced. Knee and ankle reflexes were intact, and plantar responses were flexor. There was decreased sensation to light touch and pinprick over the dorsum of the foot and anterolateral aspect of the leg.

The lesion is most likely to occur at the following root level:

A L3
B L4
C L5
D S1
E S2

3.41 A 61-year-old man in the intensive care unit had become acutely dyspnoeic and hypotensive 2 days after an aortic aneurysm repair. Apart from this operation the patient had no previous medical history and did not smoke or drink alcohol. He was still being ventilated.

On examination he appeared distressed, with intercostal recession. His skin was cold, cyanosed and clammy. His temperature was 36.5°C, pulse 110 regular and blood pressure 98/64. His respiratory rate was 26 breaths/min and there were bilateral crackles in his chest. Abdominal examination was normal. A Swan–Ganz catheter was inserted and his pulmonary artery wedge pressure was 12 mmHg. His urine output for the last 3 hours was 60 mL.

Bloods	Hb	11.5	WCC	16.7
	Neutrophils	12.8	Platelets	279
	Na	132	K	4.0
	Urea	15.7	Creatinine	176
	Protein	56	Albumin	23
	Bilirubin	16	ALT	45
	ALP	110	ESR	29
	CRP	220		

Chest X-ray	Bilateral infiltrates
	Heart size normal
ECG	Sinus tachycardia
	No ischaemic changes

Arterial blood gases on 60% O$_2$	pH	7.52	PCO$_2$	3.6
	PO$_2$	7.9	Bicarbonate	22.4
	Base excess	−2.2		

The next step in his management should be:

    A aerosolised synthetic surfactant
    B intravenous furosemide (frusemide)
    C intravenous hydrocortisone
    D putting patient prone to improve oxygenation
    E thrombolysis with TPA

3.42 A 39-year-old Caucasian man was referred because of recurrent painful ulceration of his scrotum with no associated urinary or bowel problems. He also got ulcers in his mouth. Last month he had a painful red eye that spontaneously resolved. Apart from some pain in his knee, ankle and elbow joints, which was episodic in nature, he was generally healthy. He had no previous medical history or significant family history.

On examination he has several oral and scrotal aphthous ulcers. There was some swelling and tenderness of his left knee.

Bloods	Hb	12.0	WCC	5.7
	Platelets	360	INR	1.0
	Na	134	K	4.0
	Urea	5.6	Creatinine	98
	Protein	72	Albumin	38
	Bilirubin	13	ALT	26
	ALP	60	ESR	28
	CRP	35		

Which **ONE** of the following is **NOT** associated with his condition?

A Acneiform skin eruptions
B Arterial thrombosis
C Erythema multiforme
D HLA-B5
E Pathergy

3.43 This 26-year-old HIV-positive man was admitted with headache, neck stiffness and photophobia and decreased conscious level. He was not on any medication. His temperature was 37.6°C, pulse 100 regular and blood pressure 120/88. A lumbar puncture was performed and his CSF revealed the circular opacities shown (Figure 3.43). See plate section.

The most likely organism to have caused this is:

A *Cryptococcus neoformans*
D *Listeria monocytogenes*
E *Mycobacterium tuberculosis*
F *Neisseria meningitidis*
G *Toxoplasma gondii*

3.44 A 78-year-old woman presented with pain in her back and hips. She also had decreased appetite and some loss of weight (Figure 3.44). See plate section.

The underlying diagnosis is:

A fibromyalgia
B fractured neck of femur
C multiple myeloma
D osteomalacia
E Paget's disease of bone

3.45 A 59-year-old woman was admitted with a painful, warm, swollen left leg (Figure 3.45). See plate section.

The most appropriate treatment for this patient would be:

A warfarin
B dapsone
C flucloxacillin
D indometacin
E furosemide (frusemide)

3.46 A 55-year-old man was admitted with fits. He had no history of epilepsy or head injury. He had no haemoptysis or shortness of breath but felt very tired and weak. He smoked 20 cigarettes per day for over 30 years but did not drink any alcohol. He was on no medication.

On examination he looked cachexic but there are no other abnormal findings.

Bloods				
Na	115		K	4.0
Urea	7.0		Creatinine	110
Glucose	8.0			

Thyroid and adrenal function	Normal
Urine osmolality	420 mosmol/kg
Urine Na	30 mmol/L
Chest X-ray	Coin-shaped lesion in left apex

Which ONE of the following drugs could be used to treat his condition?

A Carbamazepine
B Chlorpropamide
C Chlorothiazide
D Demeclocycline
E Vasopressin

3.47 A 60-year-old woman was brought in with acute rectal bleeding. So far today she had passed over 700 mL of fresh red blood. She had mild lower abdominal discomfort but was not vomiting. She had a previous medical history of osteoarthritis but was only taking codeine phosphate. She was not on anticoagulants. She did not drink alcohol or smoke.

On examination she was not in pain. 37.2°C, pulse 110 regular and blood pressure 95/50. Her abdomen was soft, mildly tender but there was no guarding. Bowel sounds were heard. Rectal examination revealed fresh blood but no masses.

Bloods	Hb	8.9	WCC	10.5
	Platelets	550	INR	1.1
	Na	140	K	3.9
	Urea	9.5	Creatinine	90
	Albumin	38	Protein	68
	Bilirubin	15	ALT	25
	ALP	80	Amylase	70
	Glucose	4.5		

Chest X-ray No free air under diaphragm

Abdominal X-ray No obstruction

Which of the following statements concerning diagnosis and management is true?

A An unprepared colonoscopy is the next most appropriate investigation
B Angiodysplasia is the most likely cause of bleeding
C Immediate laparotomy should be considered
D Mesenteric angiography is only useful if she continues to bleed at a rate greater than 2 mL per minute
E The source of bleeding is likely to be proximal to the ligament of Trietz

3.48 A 69-year-old man was referred because of inability to cope at home. He was able to walk with assistance. He lived alone but did not eat much; the carers complained he was persistently drooling and miserable. He had no previous medical history and had had no recent illnesses. He was not on any medication.

On examination he looked sad and did not move his head. He had a resting tremor, worsening when he tried to shake hands. His handwriting was small and illegible. He had increased tone in his upper and lower limbs. There was reduced power but in the lower limbs extensors were stronger than flexors. He had increased reflexes in the lower limbs but plantar responses were flexor. Sensation was normal. His gait was shuffling. Pupil size and fundoscopy were normal but he was unable to look down, although the other ocular movements were normal and there was no nystagmus. The other cranial nerves were normal. He had an abbreviated mental test score of 7/10. He was apyrexial, his pulse was 78 regular and his blood pressure was 120/90 sitting and standing.

The most likely diagnosis is:

A progressive supranuclear palsy/Steele–Richardson–Olszewski syndrome
B multisystem atrophy/Shy–Drager syndrome
C Huntington's disease
D Creutzfeldt–Jakob disease
E Parkinson's disease

3.49 A 60-year-old man was admitted with shortness of breath and chest pain. The symptoms had started 6 days ago but got worse today. Although known to have hypertension, he was on no medication. He did smoke but did not drink alcohol.

On examination he looked unwell and was sweating. His temperature was 36.8°C, pulse 110 regular and blood pressure 95/58 in both arms. His JVP was elevated +4 cm and both heart sounds were normal. He had decreased air entry in both lungs but there was no wheeze or crackles. His respiratory rate was 36 breaths/min. As the patient was becoming increasingly exhausted he was intubated and admitted to intensive care.

Bloods	Hb	12.9	WCC	5.8
	Platelets	256	Na	143
	K	4.2	Urea	6.1
	Creatinine	88	Protein	69
	Albumin	39	Bilirubin	14
	ALT	26	ALP	58

Chest X-ray No abnormality detected

ECG Sinus tachyardia

Arterial blood gases on 60% O_2	pH	7.28	PCO_2	6.9
	PO_2	7.6	Bicarbonate	29.1
	Base excess 3.9			

Expired CO_2 1.4

The most likely diagnosis is:

A dissection of thoracic aortic aneurysm
B inhaled foreign body
C myocardial infarction
D pneumothorax
E pulmonary embolus

3.50 A 23-year-old man with learning difficulties was referred because of dislocation of his lens. In addition he also complained of severe pain in his back and stiff joints. The joints affected included his hands, knees and spine. As a teenager he had been found to have osteoporosis and last year suffered a pulmonary embolus and was on warfarin.

On examination he was 200 cm tall. Apart from his eye condition, his fingers were long and thin, and he had pectus carinatum. His pulse was 88 regular and blood pressure 140/88. His JVP was not elevated and heart sounds were normal with no murmurs. Respiratory and abdominal examination was normal. There was some spinal tenderness as well as some inflammation of his knees and metacarpophalangeal joints. Neurological examination was normal.

Which **ONE** of the following statements concerning the diagnosis of this patient is true?

A If his urine was left to stand it would turn blue-black
B The condition cannot be diagnosed in the neonatal period
C The condition displays autosomal recessive inheritance
D The major defect is in collagen synthesis
E The most likely diagnosis is Marfan's syndrome

3.51 A 55-year-old woman was referred because of a 3-week history of jaundice and right upper quadrant pain. An ERCP was attempted but was technically difficult so a PTC was performed (Figure 3.51). See plate section.

The PTC findings are most consistent with:

A carcinoma of the head of the pancreas
B lymphoma at the porta hepatis
C pancreatic divisum
D primary sclerosing cholangitis
E stone in the common bile duct

3.52 A 73-year-old man was referred because of a painless lesion on his left lower eyelid that had been getting bigger over the past 9 months. There was no lymphadenopathy (Figure 3.52). See plate section.

The most likely diagnosis is:

A Bowen's disease
B keratoacanthoma
C nodular malignant melanoma
D basal cell carcinoma
E squamous cell carcinoma

3.53 A 17-year-old girl presented with primary amenorrhoea. She performed well at school and was a keen athlete. She had no previous medical history and was not on any medication. She did not smoke or drink alcohol.

On examination she looked well. Her height was on the 30th centile and her weight was on the 20th centile. She had breast buds but no axillary or pubic hair. She had normal female external genitalia.

Chromosome analysis	46,XX		
Bloods	17-OH Progesterone	2	(normal: <14 nmol/L)
	FSH	2.0	(normal: 2.5–10 U/L)
	LH	2.0	(normal: 2.5–10 U/L)
	Testosterone	0.8	(normal: 0.5–3.0 nmol/L)
	TSH	4	Free T$_4$ 20
Pelvic ultrasound	Normal uterus		
	Multicystic changes in the ovaries		

The most likely diagnosis is:

    A 11-β-hydroxylase deficiency
    B 5-α-reductase deficiency
    C constitutional growth delay
    D polycystic ovarian syndrome
    E primary ovarian failure

3.54 A 35-year-old woman presented with tender lesions on both legs. She had no respiratory symptoms and was not on any medication.

On examination she was apyrexial, pulse 90 regular and blood pressure 136/88. Her chest was clear. There were bilateral, erythematous raised lesions on her shins.

Chest X ray   Bihilar lymphadenopathy

The most helpful test that would give a definitive diagnosis would be:

    A Kveim test
    B serum angiotensin-converting enzyme
    C serum calcium
    D skin biopsy
    E transbronchial biopsy

3.55 A 48-year-old man presented with sudden onset right loin pain. He had no previous medical history and was not on medication (Figure 3.55). See plate section.

The likely composition of his stone is:

A calcium oxalate
B calcium phosphate
C cholesterol
D cystine
E magnesium ammonium phosphate

3.56 A 55-year-old man presented with a 2-week history of painless, frank haematuria. He reported no abdominal pain or bowel symptoms. He smoked 10 cigarettes per day but did not drink alcohol. He had no recent foreign travel and was on no medication.

On examination he was apyrexial, pulse 68 regular and blood pressure 120/70. Abdominal examination was normal and rectal examination revealed a smooth prostate.

Bloods	Hb	13.5	WCC	9.5
	Platelets	245	INR	1.1
	Na	140	K	4.2
	Urea	5.6	Creatinine	100
	Protein	68	Albumin	39
	Bilirubin	10	ALT	15
	ALP	118	ESR	15
	CRP	40		

Renal ultrasound No hydronephrosis
Left kidney 11.0 cm, right kidney 10.8 cm

Chest X-ray Normal

The most helpful test to establish the diagnosis is:

A flexible cystoscopy
B intravenous pyelogram
C prostatic specific antigen
D serum ANCA
E transrectal ultrasound

3.57 A 65-year-old man was admitted complaining of severe generalised abdominal pain, for the past 2-days, which was worse soon after eating. The pain started off colicky in nature but was now constant. Today he had also passed fresh red blood per rectum. He had a previous medical history of ischaemic heart disease and peripheral vascular disease. He was on aspirin, atenolol and digoxin. He smoked 15 cigarettes per day.

On examination he was in pain with a temperature of 37.0°C, pulse 100 irregular and blood pressure 120/70. Respiratory examination was normal. There was generalised abdominal tenderness but no guarding and no palpable masses felt. Rectal examination revealed some blood but no masses.

Bloods				
	Hb	13.5	WCC	12.5
	Platelets	300	Na	140
	K	4.0	Urea	8.5
	Creatinine	100	Albumin	35
	Protein	65	Bilirubin	12
	ALT	35	ALP	100
	GGT	60	Amylase	200
	CRP	140	ESR	35
	Lactate	5		

Arterial blood gases on air				
	pH	7.31	PCO_2	4.5
	PO_2	10.9	Bicarbonate	18
	Base excess	−7		

Chest X-ray   Normal

**Abdominal
X-ray**   Normal

The most likely diagnosis is:

  A acute diverticulitis
  B acute pancreatitis
  C bleeding from aspirin-induced gastric erosion
  D mesenteric ischaemia
  E ruptured aortic aneurysm

3.58 A 39-year-old woman was referred because of persistent hypokalaemia and hypertension going on for several months. She had no other medical problems and was treated with amlodipine and doxazosin but these had been stopped because they failed to control her hypertension. On examination her pulse was 90 and blood pressure 190/100. She was admitted overnight for tests.

Bloods	Na	140	K	2.8
	Urea	5.4	Creatinine	80

	Renin	Aldosterone
8 a.m./(lying)	0.9	1800
12 p.m./(standing)	1.2	2500

These findings are most consistent with:

    A adrenal cortex adenoma
    B adrenal medulla adenoma
    C bilateral adrenal cortical hyperplasia
    D essential hypertension
    E renal artery stenosis

3.59 A 30-year-old man was referred with a 3-month history of increasing difficulty swallowing liquids and solids. This was associated with regurgitation of food soon after eating and waking up at night coughing. His appetite was decreased and he had lost weight. He had no previous medical history and was not on any medication. Physical examination was normal.

The test that is most likely to give the definitive diagnosis is:

    A barium swallow
    B CT chest
    C endoscopic ultrasound
    D oesophageal manometery
    E upper GI endoscopy

3.60 An 80-year-old man was admitted with collapse. He reported no chest pain or shortness of breath.
    On examination his pulse was 38 regular and blood pressure 90/50. His JVP was not elevated and his heart sounds were normal. ECG showed complete heart block and a temporary pacing wire was inserted.

The postprocedure ECG (see following page) is consistent with which **ONE** of the following complications?

    A Development of acute MI
    B Electrical break
    C Electrode displacement
    D Perforation of the interventricular septum
    E Too high threshold

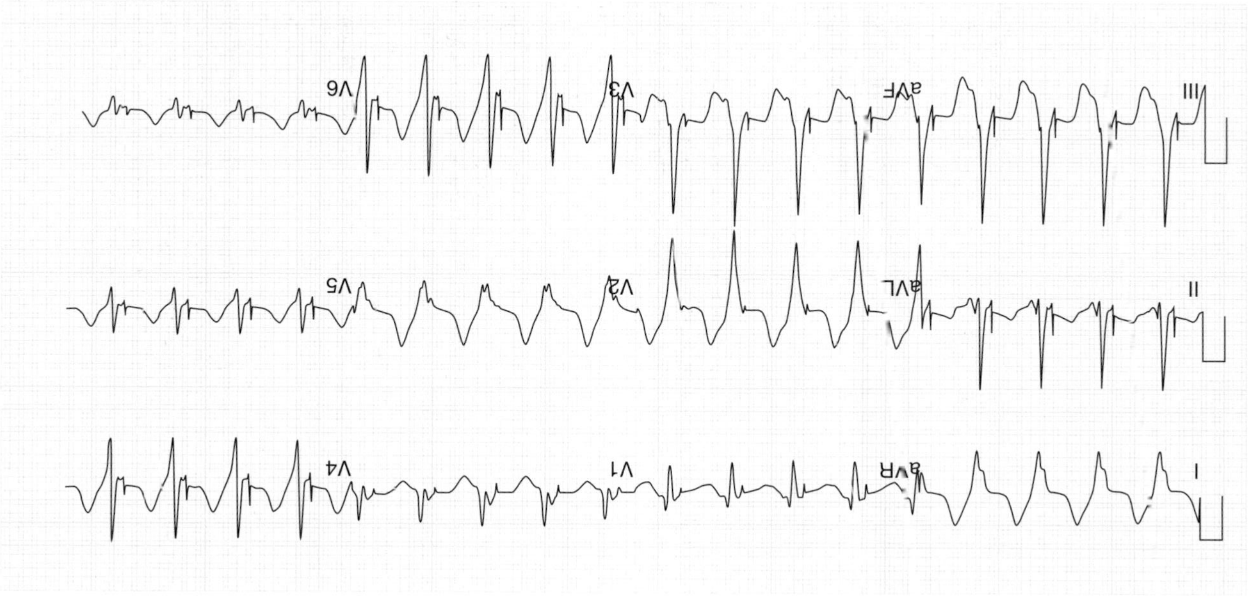
I
aVR
V1
V4
II
aVL
V2
V5
III
aVF
V3
V6

Paper 3

Answers

3.1 **A**** Contraindications to exercise testing include severe left ventricular outflow tract obstruction, severe aortic stenosis, acute myocarditis or pericarditis, left ventricular failure, unstable angina, ventricular arrhythmias, dissecting aortic aneurysm and febrile illness. LBBB may make interpretation more difficult but is not a contraindication.

3.2 **B***** The ECG shows regular P waves but occurring independently of the QRS complex, characteristic of complete heart block.

3.3 **A*** This patient has taken an overdose of insecticide, of which the commonest is an organophosphate. All these symptoms are characteristic although not specific to organophosphate poisoning. The correct treatment involves oxygen, atropine and, if necessary, pralidoxime to reactivate cholinesterase.

3.4 **D*** Orf or ecthyma contagiosum is a viral infection which begins as an inflamed reddened papule that may enlarge to form a nodule that often resolves spontaneously. It is associated with contact with infected sheep, and especially lambs. Anthrax is a bacterial infection that is associated with mild pyrexia, malaise and a malignant pustule.

3.5 **C***** An elderly man presents with headaches and bone pain. The pelvic X-ray shows thickening of the trabeculae due to bone sclerosis. All these findings are keeping with Paget's disease of bone. Other complications of Paget's disease include progressive deafness due to calcification of the ossicles and compression of cranial nerve VIII in the bony canal, blindness due to optic atrophy, a high output cardiac failure and rarely the development of osteo-sarcoma. Other bony deformities include bowing of the tibia and enlargement of the skull (see Questions 2.44 and 6.29). The main differential diagnosis would be secondary metastases. Against this possibility is the thickening of the trabeculae; myeloma and metastases usually cause lytic lesions.

3.6 **A**** The ideal study would be a cohort study, as the subjects could be grouped according to their proximity to the potentially offending source and then followed up at a later date to see if they developed brain tumours. Unfortunately this approach would be ethically unacceptable. Case control studies involve collection of data about patients with the disease and appropriate 'matched' controls without the disease, followed by comparison of the two groups regarding rates of exposure to the possible aetiological factors.

3.7   **C**** A young man presents with painless jaundice, intractable itching, hepatomegaly and previous medical history of possible inflammatory bowel disease. Stool cultures suggest no infection. The ultrasound suggests a lesion more proximal to the common bile duct. This is likely to be primary sclerosing cholangitis. This is a chronic cholestatic disease leading to progressive fibrosis of the intra- and extrahepatic bile ducts, which can lead to secondary biliary cirrhosis and ultimately hepatic failure. ERCP is the gold standard for diagnosing primary sclerosing cholangitis, showing strictures and a beading pattern, which may not be detected by MRCP.

3.8   **D**** A teenager presents with abdominal pain, jaundice, macrocytic anaemia and increased urinary urobilinogen and is Coombs' test/direct antiglobulin test negative. The most likely diagnosis is hereditary spherocytosis. This is a form of hereditary intravascular haemolysis where there is a defect in red cell membrane spectrin so that all are spherical in shape, as opposed to being biconcave discs. The spleen recognises them as abnormal and causes their destruction. Clinical sequelae include anaemia, splenomegaly, leg ulcers and pigment gallstones. Biochemical tests show a raised serum (unconjugated) bilirubin. The Coombs' test is negative and therefore excludes an auto-immune haemolytic anaemia. Osmotic fragility studies will confirm the diagnosis. When red cells are placed in hypotonic solution they swell up and lyse; this is more so with spherocytes. Ham's test is a test for paroxysmal nocturnal haemoglobinuria. Schumm's test is a test for the presence of methaemalbumin.

3.9   **C**** The histology slide shows the *Giardia lamblia* flagellate protozoa between the villi. None of the options would give such a picture. Although giardiasis is often associated with foreign travel, it must always be considered in all cases of chronic diarrhoea.

3.10 **B*** Dengue fever begins with symptoms of an upper respiratory tract infection. To diagnose dengue haemorrhagic fever there needs to be fever of recent onset; haemorrhagic manifestations, in this case epistaxis, microscopic haematuria, haematemesis and melaena; low platelet count; and evidence of leaky capillaries, in this case albumin <30. There is no available vaccination and treatment is symptomatic. Yellow fever is another viral haemorrhagic fever and has similar clinical features but is found only in Africa and South America and a vaccination is available. Hepatitis A is unlikely as the incubation period is normally 2 weeks and would be associated with more deranged transaminases in a patient this unwell. Typhoid and blackwater fever are discussed in another question (see 1.11).

3.11 **E*** The insidious onset symptoms of proximal myopathy with no evidence of nerve involvement are likely to be a form of primary muscle disease. Patients with limb–girdle muscular dystrophy tend to have severe disability much earlier on, i.e. early twenties. Polymyalgia rheumatica does not cause cardiac or swallowing problems, although both are associated with elevated ESR and possibly muscle tenderness. Serum creatine kinase levels, electromyography and muscle biopsy can be used to confirm the diagnosis. The loss of weight, anorexia, dysphagia and atrial fibrillation suggest there may be an underlying oesophageal carcinoma.

3.12 A** There is a large, dark, pigmented mass that is emerging nasal to the optic disc and appears to be invading the optic nerve. This appearance would be consistent with a choroidal (below the retina) melanoma. A choroidal melanoma would not cause blurred vision, unless it encroached on the macula, in which case it might cause a field defect.

3.13 G, I* From the lung function tests, the patient has a restrictive lung defect, as shown by a FEV_1: FVC ratio of 75% and a reduced TLC. The TLCO is the transfer factor and gives an indication of how easy it is for gas to cross the alveolar lining. In restrictive disease this value is decreased. The KCO is very similar to the TLCO but now takes into account the effective surface area of the diffusion area. Causes of increased KCO include pulmonary haemorrhage, arteriovenous shunts, asthma and removal of non-functioning lung. The discrepancy between a reduced TLCO and normal KCO would be explained by pulmonary haemorrhage and removal of an effectively dead part of lung.

3.14 A** This woman has the signs and symptoms of a bilateral symmetrical arthritis consistent with rheumatoid arthritis. While prognosis is very variable, certain markers are associated with more severe disease: positive rheumatoid factor; presence of extra-articular features especially nodules and vasculitis; HLA-DR4 genetic marker; female sex; radiographic erosions within 2 years of disease onset; and severe disability at presentation. Insidious onset of the arthritis is also associated with more severe disease as opposed to palindromic rheumatism, which is characterised by episodic attacks followed by complete resolution in between.

3.15 B*** This patient has frontal balding, wasting of the facial, shoulder and temporalis muscles, and bilateral ptosis. All of these could be explained by dystrophia myotonica (see **2.46**).

3.16 A*** This barium enema shows an 'apple core' lesion in the distal transverse colon. This should be treated as a colonic neoplasm until proven otherwise, even though the stricture is relatively smooth and there is no soft tissue shadow of an obstructing carcinoma. There are some isolated diverticula but these are not the most salient feature of this X-ray.

3.17 A** This ERCP shows a common bile duct, which is narrow distally and dilated proximally. This would be consistent with compression of the common bile duct by a pancreatic neoplasm. There are no gallstones.

3.18 E* For explanation of how to interpret cardiac catheterisation values see **2.19**. There is an increase in the oxygen saturation between the right atrium and right ventricle. This suggests that there is a ventricular septal defect, as oxygenated blood from the left ventricle is mixing with the deoxygenated blood of the right ventricle.

3.19 C* After complex 3 on the ECG trace the R wave of complex 4 coincides with the T wave of complex 3, the so-called 'R-on-T phenomenon'. Following this there is a regular but sinusoidal broad complex tachycardia that is characteristic of torsades de pointes and he is still maintaining a pulse.

3.20 A* If patients with methanol poisoning are admitted within 1 hour of ingestion then gastric lavage could be attempted. Activated charcoal does not adsorb methanol and ipecacuanha is contraindicated because of the risk of aspiration. The metabolic acidosis is corrected with intravenous sodium bicarbonate to keep the pH >7.20. Indications for haemodialysis or peritoneal dialysis include: presence of mental or visual features; plasma methanol concentration >500 mg/L; and worsening acidosis not responding to intravenous bicarbonate.

3.21 B* This patient has a symmetrical erythematous rash affecting both upper and lower limbs and also affecting the mouth. The diagnosis is erythema multiforme. The rash may be due to penicillin or mycoplasma pneumonia.

3.22 C* This patient appears to be having a myxoedematous crisis. Certainly thyroxine or T_3 should be given, albeit in small quantities. Such patients may have other endocrine problems, for example adrenal failure, and no harm could come from assuming she may be Addisonian and treating her with steroids. She needs rewarming and antibiotics in case there is an underlying infection. Lugol's iodine solution is used to treat thyrotoxicosis.

3.23 B* RR is the ratio of the incidence of death in the exposed group (i.e. smokers) to the incidence of death in the non-exposed group (non-smokers).

Incidence among smokers = 10/100

Incidence among non-smokers = 20/300

RR = (10/100)/(20/300) = (10 × 300)/(20 × 100) = 1.5

As the RR >1, this would suggest a positive association between smoking and death.

	Dead	Alive	
Smoker	10	90	100
Non-smoker	20	280	300
	30	370	400

3.24 A** Blood results show elevated autoantibodies and a raised globulin (protein − albumin = 42) consistent with autoimmune hepatitis. There are three main types of autoimmune hepatitis. Type I is associated with elevated antinuclear antibodies and smooth muscle antibodies. To be clinically significant these titres ought to be greater than 1 in 80. Type II is associated with elevated anti-LKM (anti-liver–kidney–muscle antibodies); this form is more associated with other autoimmune conditions such as insulin dependent diabetes, autoimmune thyroiditis and vitiligo. Type III is the least prevalent form and is more associated with antibodies to soluble liver antigen/liver–pancreas (anti-SLA/LP). Liver biopsy typically shows an interface hepatitis with disruption of the limiting plate of the portal tract. The antimitochondrial antibody titre is not significant and is not diagnostic of primary biliary cirrhosis. There are no features of systemic lupus erythematosus and she is anti-double stranded DNA negative. The normal caeruloplasmin goes against Wilson's disease.

3.25 E** This patient presents with pyrexia, chest tightness, shock and haemoglobinuria, which are consistent with an acute haemolytic transfusion reaction probably due to ABO incompatibility or bacterial contamination of the blood unit being transfused. Treatment would involve stopping the transfusion, fluid resuscitation and informing the blood bank of the reaction.

3.26 B** All of the options could cause small bowel obstruction. The slide shows islands of uniform cells, which are not mitotic and without lots of nuclei that would suggest adenocarcinoma. Synaptophysin stains for neuroendocrine tumours and stains the cytoplasm brown. With ischaemic bowel there is normal structure but with a pink, necrotic epithelium; as the ischaemia worsens so does the necrosis as it spreads towards the serosa where it can perforate.

3.27 A** The long history of a flu-like illness, night sweats, pyrexia, cervical lymphadenopathy and hepatosplenomegaly after visiting a Mediterranean country is suggestive of brucellosis. The patient may have handled cattle or ingested unpasteurised dairy products. Lymphoma is a possibility but Hodgkin's disease would be more likely if there was associated eosinophilia and pruritus in an older person. Leishmaniasis is another possible differential diagnosis.

3.28 E* This patient has primary polydipsia. No mention was made of the urine volume produced but it is likely to be greater than 4 litres. The urine osmolality is greater than 300 mosmol/kg, thereby suggesting this is not diabetes insipidus. The urine becomes more concentrated as the patient is more water deprived. There is only a modest increase in the urine osmolality with DDAVP (desmopressin) injection. In a normal person one would expect the urine osmolality to be >750 mosmol/kg but due to chronic polydipsia and polyuria there is a reduction in the concentrating power of the nephron, due to the washout of solute from the renal interstitium. Partial nephrogenic diabetes insipidus would produce a similar water deprivation test but there would be a higher than normal plasma$_{ADH}$ level.

3.29 D** Of all the responses only a pulmonary embolus is likely to cause a respiratory alkalosis in a hypoxic patient. A salicylate overdose may cause respiratory alkalosis compensating for the metabolic acidosis but for that to occur over 24 hours post ingestion would be unusual.

3.30 E*** The most likely diagnosis in this patient is temporal or giant cell arteritis. A properly performed biopsy will define the need for therapy in 85% of cases but because the arteritis is patchy, biopsy may miss the area of inflammation. If the clinical condition warranted it, high dose prednisolone should be started before the biopsy is taken to prevent blindness.

3.31 C** The history is of a patient who has a long history of erratic bowel movements. Frequent overuse of laxatives, especially those which are anthracine-derived, can result in generalised pigmentation of the bowel when viewed endoscopically. No treatment is required.

3.32 E** This patient has had a thoracoplasty as collapse therapy for tuberculosis involving the upper six ribs on the right. The chest wall is deformed because of the surgery performed. There is fibrosis in the right apex and left apical and basal regions; a recrudescence of TB is a possibility that must always be considered, particularly if he was not treated with anti-TB drugs.

3.33 C** This patient has a history of recent foreign travel, cough, gastrointestinal symptoms, deranged liver function tests and right upper lobe pneumonia. The most likely diagnosis is legionnaire's disease. The most appropriate antibiotics would be an intravenous macrolide and rifampicin. The chest X-ray appearances of legionnaire's disease can vary widely from a ground-glass appearance to a peripheral lobar consolidation.

3.34 D** This young woman presents with fever, confusion, Janeway lesions on her hands, and a murmur. The murmur could be due to a floppy mitral valve prolapse that had infective vegetations, which were embolising to the brain making infective endocarditis a very real possibility. She does not have any signs or symptoms of meningitis. Encephalitis presents with altered consciousness, personality changes, seizures, and paresis and cranial nerve involvement. There is nothing in the history to suggest toxic shock syndrome.

3.35 E** The ECG shows broad complex tachycardia, concordance of the chest leads (deep S waves in V_{1-6}), right axis deviation, fusion beat (beat 9) on the rhythm strip and dissociated P waves (see V_5). Fusion beats occur when a supraventricular impulse and an impulse originating from the ventricle depolarise the ventricle simultaneously and resemble a combination of the two beats. Dissociated P waves or independent P wave activity is another characteristic of VT; if they were retrograde P waves, they would look morphologically the same, but in this case the P waves appear to be 'buried' within the QRS complex. Other characteristics of VT include: capture beats, QRS complex >140 ms, ventricular rate >160 beats/min, atypical right bundle branch block and history of ischaemic heart disease.

3.36 A*** This patient is likely to suffer from a number of conditions like sarcoidosis or secondary to various drugs. The differential diagnosis for this lesion includes pretibial myxoedema, which would be expected to have a raised *peau d'orange* appearance.

3.37 D** This patient has a pituitary tumour. It is possible that it will grow inferiorly to involve the cavernous sinus. Within the cavernous sinus run the internal carotid artery, oculomotor, trochlear, abducens and ophthalmic and maxillary branches of the trigeminal nerve. The mandibular branch of the trigeminal nerve supplies sensation to the lower face and anterior two-thirds of the tongue.

3.38 D** Although this patient was not able to communicate verbally, he understood his condition. The principle of autonomy dictates that he can decide what treatment he wants. Oral feeding and drinking constitute basic care. Nasogastric tubes, intravenous fluids, artificial feeding and PEG insertion are considered treatments; if a patient refuses these, that is his prerogative and he can choose not to have them, even though he may die without them.

3.39 C** A young boy presents with abdominal pain and jaundice of short duration. The only abnormal blood result is the raised bilirubin. An ALP <785 in 13-year-old boys is normal and represents adolescent bone growth. Gilbert's syndrome is an asymptomatic congenital hyperbilirubinaemia characterised by a deficiency of bilirubin glucuronidase leading to unconjugated hyperbilirubinaemia. The condition can present itself during times of intercurrent illness, vomiting or fasting. There is no treatment. Diagnosis can be confirmed by finding raised serum levels of unconjugated bilirubin and normal reticulocyte count to distinguish it from haemolysis. With hereditary spherocytosis, the clinical picture may be very similar but often patients have splenomegaly. Dubin–Johnson syndrome is a benign autosomal recessive (AR) condition causing conjugated hyperbilirubinaemia due to defective excretion of bile into the canaliculi. There is no alteration of liver enzymes except raised serum levels of conjugated bilirubin; on liver biopsy the colour is green-black but of normal architecture. Rotor syndrome is another benign AR condition due to defective uptake and storage of organic acids in the liver resulting in conjugated hyperbilirubinaemia; liver biopsy is normal. Biliary atresia is progressive inflammation of the biliary tree leading to a failure to excrete bile which leads to scarring and cirrhosis. Treatment is surgical and may need transplantation.

3.40 C** This could have occurred as a result of a prolapsed intervertebral disc. The most common radiculopathies involve roots L4, L5 and S1. L5 lesions involve the toe extensors. Lesions to L3 and L4 would involve the knee jerk. Lesions to S1 would involve the ankle jerk and the plantar flexors. S2 lesions would not result in muscle weakness but may involve the ankle jerk and sensation in the perianal region.

3.41 D* This patient's acute deterioration is most likely to be due to ARDS, an acute syndrome caused by direct or indirect injury to the lung. The exact pathogenesis is unknown but it may be triggered by a number of events, including sepsis, blood transfusions, chest trauma and aspiration of gastric contents. According to the American-European Consensus Conference, to diagnose ARDS three criteria need to be met: (1) new infiltrates on chest X-ray; (2) PAWP ≤ 18 mmHg, i.e. non-cardiogenic pulmonary oedema (3) P_aO_2/FiO_2 (arterial oxygen partial pressure: inhaled oxygen) ratio greater than 200 mmHg or 40 kPa. In this case the patient is oliguric, has a low PAWP and is hypotensive so the main principle of treatment is to ensure he is well filled; diuresis is likely to cause intravascular depletion and worsen renal failure. Unlike neonatal respiratory distress syndrome, neither surfactant nor steroids have been shown to improve prognosis of ARDS. There is thought to be an element of right-to-left shunting through atelectatic and consolidated lung units that are not ventilated. Turning patients prone can shift perfusion to previously non-ventilated lung zones.

3.42 C* This patient has Behçet's syndrome, which is a vasculitis that is characterised by recurrent orogenital ulceration, eye lesions, arthritis and skin lesions. The skin lesions include erythema nodosum, thrombophlebitis, acneiform skin eruption and hyperirritability of the skin (pathergy). The condition is more prevalent from the Eastern Mediterranean and Turkey to the Far East and there is an association with HLA-B5 and B51 not B27. Twenty-five per cent of patients may develop arterial or venous thrombosis, which may lead to the formation of aneurysms. Up to a third of these patients have factor V Leiden mutation.

3.43 A** This patient has meningitis secondary to *C. neoformans*. The CSF has been stained with Indian ink and shows the characteristic haloes of *C. neoformans*. The patient should be treated with amphotericin.

3.44 D* This pelvic X-ray shows pseudofractures or 'Looser's zones' in the neck of both femurs. They are characteristic of osteomalacia.

3.45 B** This patient appears to have left lower limb cellulitis. The correct management involves antibiotics against *Staphylococcus aureus*, such as flucloxacillin.

3.46 D** This patient has a serum osmolality of 253 mosmol/kg (serum osmolality = 2× ([Na] + [K]) + [urea] + [glucose]). He has SIADH, as shown by a low serum osmolality, normal concentration of his urine, dilutional hyponatraemia and a probable lung neoplasm. To fully diagnose SIADH, patients have to be euvolaemic, have normal thyroid, renal and adrenal function tests and a urinary Na > 20 mmol/L. The normal treatment of SIADH and hyponatraemia is fluid restriction. However, should that fail, then possible treatments include demeclocycline or lithium. Fits in this case should be treated with phenytoin.

3.47 D** A patient presents with large volume, fresh, red, rectal bleeding. The next most appropriate test after resuscitating her would be a prepared colonoscopy. Usually a phosphate enema can be given, otherwise blood and faeces are likely to obstruct the view. Diverticular disease or even neoplasms are more likely than angiodysplasia of the colon. For angiography to detect a lesion there needs to be active bleeding. Bleeding proximal to the ligament of Trietz is likely to present as melaena rather than red blood per rectum.

3.48 A* This patient has Parkinson's syndrome with pyramidal features, thereby making it a Parkinson's plus syndrome. There is no autonomic involvement, which goes against multisystem atrophy. There is a problem with the supranuclear connections of the oculomotor nerve leading to vertical conjugate gaze palsy. Parinaud's syndrome involves damage to the midbrain and superior colliculus, resulting in loss of the light reflex, retraction of the eyelids and relative mydriasis.

3.49 E** This patient presents as having had a massive central pulmonary embolism. This is why his arterial PO_2 and PCO_2 are low and consistent with a type I respiratory failure pattern. His expired CO_2 is low because the embolism has managed to block the pulmonary artery and therefore very little air with CO_2 is being expired.

3.50 C** Tall stature, downward dislocation of the lens, mental retardation, chest wall deformity, arachnodactyly and evidence of thromboembolism are all features of homocystinuria. This is an autosomal recessive disorder due to deficiency of cystathione b-synthase, leading to increased homocystine in the blood and urine. Newborn homocystine screening is available. Alkaptonuria is associated with urine that turns blue-black on standing. Marfan's syndrome is an autosomal dominant disease of type I collagen and is associated with upward dislocation of the lens and aortic dissection but not thrombo-embolism or mental retardation.

3.51 E** The scan shows dilated intrahepatic ducts and common bile duct, suggesting a proximal biliary lesion. There is some beading of the intrahepatic ducts but not characteristic of sclerosing cholangitis. There are stones in the distal common bile duct and obstructing the proximal common bile duct.

3.52 D*** There is a crateriform ulcer on the lower lid with a raised, pearly and telangiectatic edge and crusty surface. Basal cell carcinomas hardly ever metastasise but instead cause local infiltration and destruction. Squamous cell carcinomas start off as warty, hyperkeratotic nodules, which can ulcerate and typically have everted edges. They are usually faster growing and can metastasise via the lymph nodes. Keratoacanthomas are benign, rapidly growing tumours that are characterised by having a central horny plug and may resolve spontaneously. Bowen's disease is a form of superficial squamous cell carcinoma in situ that presents as psoriasis-like or eczema-like lesion.

3.53 C** Primary amenorrhoea is defined as no menses by age 16. Extremely active girls like runners, swimmers, gymnasts and ballet dancers are well known to undergo delayed puberty and menarche. Her pelvic ultrasound showed normal internal genitalia, albeit with multiple cysts on her ovaries, and this is normal for a girl of her age. With polycystic ovarian syndrome one would expect her to be obese and have raised LH and testosterone levels. She has normal external genitalia, thereby excluding 5-α-reductase deficiency and 11-β-hydroxylase deficiency.

3.54 E** Bihilar lymphadenopathy and erythema nodosum is highly suggestive of sarcoidosis. Serum ACE would be positive in >70% patients but would also be positive with TB, lymphoma, asbestosis and silicosis. Serum calcium is raised in >60% but is not specific. Transbronchial biopsy would show infiltration of the alveolar walls and interstitial spaces, with inflammatory cells and granuloma formation in >90% even in cases where the chest X-ray shows no parenchymal involvement, thereby giving a histological diagnosis. The Kveim test is no longer performed because of the potential risk of transmitting HIV or other prion diseases.

3.55 E** This patient has a 'staghorn' calculus. The most likely composition of these types of stones is 'struvite', which contains magnesium ammonium phosphate and sometimes calcium associated with infection.

3.56 A*** Patients with unexplained painless haematuria need to undergo cystoscopy to exclude a bladder carcinoma.

3.57 D** This patient is an arteriopath, has a history of atrial fibrillation and presents with abdominal pain that is worse after eating, which would be most consistent with mesenteric ischaemia. Patients may often present with vague abdominal symptoms and minimal abdominal findings. The raised lactate is suggestive of ischaemia, which would be unusual in someone with diverticulitis unless perforation had occurred. CT abdomen and/or mesenteric angiography would be the investigations of choice. Abdominal X-ray may show bowel wall thickening or thumb printing, although this may not present acutely.

3.58 C* This patient has Conn's syndrome, as shown by low baseline serum renin and elevated serum aldosterone. The patient is admitted for overnight lying and standing renin and aldosterone measurements to differentiate between adrenal cortex adenoma and adrenocortical hyperplasia. When patients with Conn's syndrome are lying down, the serum aldosterone is high and the serum renin is high. When patients stand up and have been ambulating there is an increase in the serum renin. With patients who have adrenal cortical hyperplasia, there is an increase in serum aldosterone after standing because the tissue is still stimulated by renin; patients with adrenal cortex adenomas have a decreased serum aldosterone because the tumour is unresponsive to renin. ACTH stimulates adrenal cortex adenomas; this follows a diurnal variation and is decreased during the day.

3.59 D** A young man with progressive dysphagia, regurgitation and nocturnal cough is most likely to have achalasia. Oesophageal manometry is the 'gold standard' for early diagnosis of the condition and will show failure of the lower oesophageal sphincter to relax, lack of peristalsis and elevated lower oesophageal sphincter pressure. Upper GI endoscopy may show a large dilated oesophagus later. In practice, upper GI endoscopy would be done to exclude 'pseudoachalasia' usually due to a tumour below the gastro-oesophageal junction. A barium swallow can be useful in detecting achalasia and does produce a characteristic picture (see 1.18) but only in a proportion of patients.

3.60 D* The ECG shows a normal electrical capture as each pacing spike is followed by a QRS complex. Normally there should be LBBB following insertion of the pacing wire. In this case there is RBBB suggestive of perforation of the interventricular septum and pacing of the left ventricle.

Paper 4

Questions

4.1 A 55-year-old man was noted by his general practitioner to have atrial fibrillation. He had no other medical problems and was not on any medication. He drank alcohol occasionally.

His pulse was 80 irregular and blood pressure 130/78. His JVP was not elevated and his heart sounds and chest were normal.

Bloods				
	Hb	13.8	WCC	6.6
	Platelets	230	Na	140
	K	4.5	Urea	4.2
	Creatinine	89	Magnesium	0.80
	Calcium	2.30	Glucose	4.3
	TSH	2.2	Free T$_4$	14.6

This patient should be treated with:

A amiodarone
B aspirin
C digoxin
D sotalol
E warfarin

4.2 A 69-year-old man was admitted with dizziness.

His ECG shows:

A 1st degree AV block
B complete heart block
C Mobitz type I 2nd degree AV block
D Mobitz type II 2nd degree AV block
E sinus bradycardia

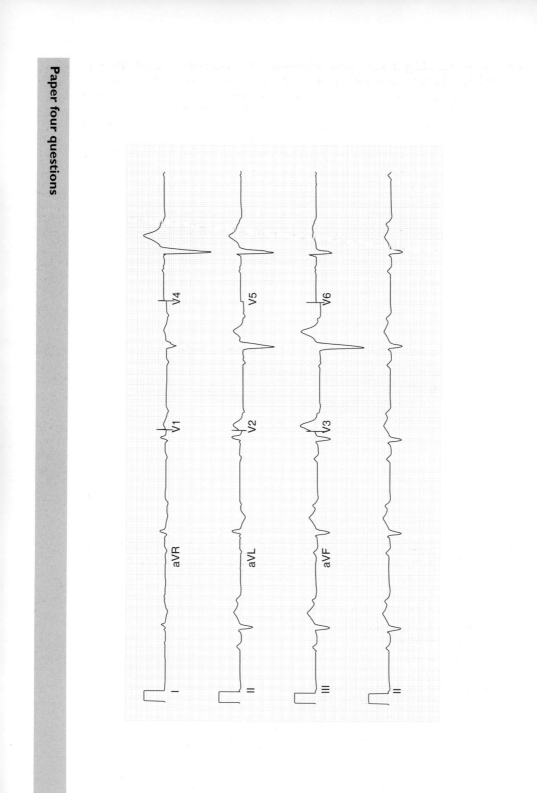

4.3 A 16-year-old girl was found collapsed in the toilet of the ward. She was admitted 3 days ago with a paracetamol overdose from which she was making a good recovery. The nursing staff suspected that she had taken another overdose of another drug. The patient complained of dizziness.

On examination she was alert. Her temperature was 37.0°C, pulse 40 regular and blood pressure 78/40. JVP was not elevated and both heart sounds were present. Her respiratory rate was 26 breaths per minute and chest was clear. Abdominal examination was normal. Her pupils were dilated.

Bloods	Hb	13.2	WCC	9.9
	Platelets	340	INR	1.0
	Na	135	K	4.0
	U	3.8	Creatinine	88
	Protein	70	Albumin	39
	Bilirubin	15	ALT	50
	ALP	100	Calcium	2.22
	Magnesium	0.72		
ECG	1st degree AV block		Heart rate 40	

The most likely overdose this patient has taken is:

A amitriptyline
B atenolol
C codeine phosphate
D diazepam
E digoxin

4.4 A 16-year-old girl developed a mild fever and a lesion around her mouth 4 days ago. She was not on any medication (Figure 4.4). See plate section.

The most likely diagnosis is:

A impetigo contagiosa
B gingivostomatitis
C tinea capitis
D seborrhoeic dermatitis
E rosacea

4.5 A 16-year-old boy presented with a 1-week history of cough, abdominal pain and weight loss. He had recently returned from visiting his family in Pakistan.

On examination he was apyrexial and not jaundiced. Pulse was 90 regular and blood pressure 100/60. His chest was clear but he had some mild generalised abdominal tenderness.

Bloods	Hb	13.4	WCC	9.8
	Platelets	269	Na	127
	K	6.1	Urea	8.5
	Creatinine	90	Glucose	3.0
	Calcium	2.88	Phosphate	1.1
	Amylase	80		

Blood gases on air	pH	7.31	PCO_2	3.7
	PO_2	10.6	Bicarbonate	18

Urine osmolality 320 mosmol/kg

The most likely diagnosis is:

    A Addison's disease
    B Cushing's syndrome
    C Diabetes insipidus
    D Nelson's disease
    E SIADH

4.6 The research and development committee at the university have to consider applications for research. A number of proposals, all claiming to be randomised control trials (RCTs) have been submitted. You have been asked to determine which of the proposals' study designs is most appropriate for an RCT.

Which **ONE** of the following would be most appropriate for a RCT?

    A Whether atenolol can prevent recurrence of stroke
    B Whether glucosuria can predict diabetes mellitus
    C Whether hypertension is associated with chronic renal failure
    D Whether hypertriglyceridaemia is associated with acute pancreatitis
    E Whether smoking during pregnancy increases fetal loss

4.7 A 49-year-old man presented with a 1-week history of persistent dull upper abdominal pain and fever. He also complained of pale stools and episodic dark urine. He had decreased appetite, some weight loss and looked yellow. Eighteen months earlier he had undergone laparoscopic cholecystectomy for gallstones, and ERCP 4 months ago to remove sludge from the common bile duct. He drank 10 units of alcohol per week and smoked 15 cigarettes per day. He was not on any medication.

On examination he was jaundiced, had a temperature of 39.1°C, pulse 120 regular and blood pressure 120/60. There was right upper quadrant abdominal tenderness but no hepatosplenomegaly and no ascites. Rectal examination was normal. He was not encephalopathic.

Bloods

Hb	12.5	WCC	15.6
Platelets	345	INR	1.5
Na	136	K	4.5
Urea	5.9	Creatinine	120
Bilirubin	62	Albumin	30
Protein	60	AST	60
ALP	360	GGT	140

Chest X-ray Normal

Urinalysis Bilirubin 1+, no urobilinogen, no protein, no white cells

The test that would ascertain the diagnosis would be:

A Alpha-fetoprotein
B blood culture
C CT abdomen
D ERCP
E liver biopsy

4.8 A 60-year-old man was referred because of pruritus, headache and hypertension. He had no previous medical history and was on no medication.

On examination he had a plethoric face. His temperature was 37.0°C, pulse 88 regular and blood pressure 165/90. JVP was elevated to +4 cm and both heart sounds were normal. His chest was clear. Abdominal examination was normal except for a palpable spleen.

Bloods

Hb	18.5	MCV	99.2
WCC	10.6	Platelets	600
Haematocrit	56%	Red cell mass	36 mL/kg
Neutrophils	7.2	Lymphocytes	3.1
Monocytes	0.3	Na	135
K	4.0	Urea	5.3
Creatinine	88		

Which **ONE** of the following would be consistent with a diagnosis of poly-cythaemia rubra vera?

A Enlarged kidneys on ultrasound
B Low neutrophil alkaline phosphatase score
C Low serum erythropoietin
D O_2 saturation on air <92%
E Packed cell volume <0.40

4.9 A 58-year-old Pakistani man was admitted with shortness of breath associated with a dry cough. His appetite was decreased and he had lost weight. He smoked 20 cigarettes a day for the last 35 years. He had a previous medical history of pulmonary TB, which had affected the right apical region, and he had completed a course of anti-TB medication. He was on no medication.

On examination he was cachexic. His temperature was 37.0°C, pulse 88 regular, blood pressure 140/88 and respiratory rate 20 breaths/min. He had decreased air entry and breath sounds on the right lung.

Chest X-ray	See Figure 4.9 in plate section.
Biopsy of right lung lesion	(Plate 4.9). See plate section.

The most likely diagnosis is:

A *Pneumocystis carinii* pneumonia
B pulmonary TB
C carcinoma of the lung
D *Aspergillus sp.* infection
E sarcoidosis

4.10 A 35-year-old hepatitis C-positive man was referred for treatment. He was an ex-intravenous drug user who had stopped abusing drugs 3 years ago; he was hepatitis B-negative and HIV-negative. He complained of arthralgia and abdominal discomfort. He had no other medical or psychiatric problems. He drank 2 units of alcohol per week and smoked 15 cigarettes per day.

Bloods				
	Hb	14.5	WCC	5.5
	Platelets	85	INR	1.0
	Protein	72	Albumin	35
	Bilirubin	15	ALT	70
	ALP	100	GGT	95
	Alpha-fetoprotein	5		

HCV PCR RNA Positive

HCV genotype 1

Liver ultrasound Liver normal sized with no focal lesion.

Normal blood flow, intrahepatic ducts and common bile duct

Liver biopsy Moderate active fibrosis

No cirrhosis

The best management plan for this patient is:

A azathioprine
B lamivudine
C observe and repeat blood tests in 3 months time
D prednisolone
E ribavirin and α-interferon

4.11 A 35-year-old woman presented with progressive fatigue and weakness. She had had to give up work as a secretary because her hands became uncomfortable after a short period of typing. However, there was no paresthesiae and her symptoms improved with rest. She also complained of some double vision, dysphagia and shortness of breath on exertion. Three years ago hypothyroidism and type 1 diabetes was diagnosed but she had good control and regular follow-up at the diabetic clinic. She has had no recent illnesses.

On examination she had bilateral ptosis and strabismus. The rest of her cranial nerve examination was normal. Her pulse was 72 regular and blood pressure 120/80. Respiratory examination was normal. There was no limb muscle wasting or weakness. Tone, power, reflexes and sensation were normal, as was neck examination.

The most likely diagnosis is:

A dystrophia myotonica
B myasthenia gravis
C Eaton–Lambert syndrome
D motor neurone disease
E mononeuritis multiplex

4.12 A 42-year-old woman was referred with headaches. As part of the examination, fundoscopy was performed and is shown below (Figure 4.12). See plate section.

The fundoscopic appearance is most likely due to:

A coloboma
B neovascularisation
C myelinated fibres
D optic atrophy
E swollen optic disc

4.13 A previously well 25-year-old woman presented with 2-day history of cough productive of green purulent sputum. She had no allergies and did not keep any pets. She had not been abroad and had not come into contact with anyone else who had an illness. She had a normal appetite and no weight loss.

On examination she had a temperature of 37.4°C. Her pulse was 90 regular, blood pressure 120/75 and her respiratory rate was 20 breaths/min. There were crackles and bronchial breathing in the right mid-zone.

Bloods

Hb	14.5	WCC	14.5
Neutrophils	11.3	Platelets	270
Na	139	K	4.5
Urea	4.5	Creatinine	86
Protein	70	Albumin	38
Bilirubin	10	ALT	20
ALP	69	CRP	45

Chest X-ray Consolidation in the right midzone

The best antibiotic treatment for this patient is:

   A amoxicillin and clarithromycin
   B ciprofloxacin and gentamicin
   C clarithromycin and metronidazole
   D rifampicin and clarthromycin
   E rifampicin, isoniazid and pyrazinamide

4.14 A 26-year-old woman presented with fever, shortness of breath and joint pain. Her symptoms had started 2 weeks ago but lethargy and weakness were increasing. She had right pleuritic chest pain; she had not been on any long-haul flights, nor had any periods of immobility and was not on the oral contraceptive pill. Previously she had normal exercise tolerance. The joints affected included both wrists and metacarpophalangeal joints, which were inflamed, swollen and tender. She had noticed blood in her urine for the past 3 days but no associated abdominal pain. Her last menstrual period was 2 weeks ago. Recently she had developed a rash on her scalp that took some months to improve but had left her with scarring and alopecia. She was on no medication. She smoked 15 cigarettes per day.

On examination she had a temperature of 38.0°C, pulse 96 regular and blood pressure 150/98. Cardiovascular examination was normal but on auscultation of her chest there was a right pleural rub. Abdominal examination was normal. Apart from her hands, all other joints were normal.

Bloods				
	Hb	11.7	MCV	92.2
	WCC	2.66	Neutrophils	2.0
	Lymphocytes	0.6	Eosinophils	0.06
	Platelets	170	Na	138
	K	4.2	Urea	9.8
	Creatinine	130	Protein	70
	Albumin	34	Bilirubin	12
	ALT	19	ALP	79
	Creatinine kinase	100	ESR	38
	CRP	5	C3	0.45
	C4	0.10		

Rheumatoid factor Negative

Antinuclear antibody 1 in 80

Anti-Sm antibody 1 in 40

Anti-Ro antibody Negative

Anti-La antibody Negative

c-ANCA Negative

Urine dipstick Blood 2+, protein 3+

Chest X-ray Normal

Hand X-ray Soft tissue swelling around wrist and metacarpophalangeal joints

The most likely diagnosis is:

    A Churg–Strauss syndrome
    B mixed connective tissue disease
    C polyarteritis nodosa
    D rheumatoid arthritis
    E systemic lupus erythematosus

4.15 This 56-year-old women was referred complaining of lethargy (Figure 4.15). See plate section.

The most likely diagnosis is:

    A acromegaly
    B Cushing's syndrome
    C hypopituitarism
    D hypothyroidism
    E Paget's disease

4.16 A 79-year-old woman known to suffer from hypertension and on warfarin for atrial fibrillation was admitted with right hemiparesis and aphasia. There was no history of trauma (Figure 4.16). See plate section.

The CT scan (Figure 4.16) shows:

A left cerebral infarct
B left extradural haematoma
C left intracerebral haemorrhage
D left subdural haematoma
E subarachnoid haemorrhage

4.17 A 61-year-old woman was referred with a 5-week history of progressive dysphagia and weight loss (Figure 4.17). See plate section.

The most likely diagnosis is:

A achalasia
B benign stricture
C carcinoma of the oesophagus
D oesophageal candidiasis
E oesophageal varices

4.18 A 60-year-old man was referred for cardiac catheterisation because of progressive shortness of breath and the presence of a murmur.

| | Pressure | Normal value | O_2 saturation |
	(systolic/diastolic/mmHg)		(%)
Right atrium (mean)	8	0–8	73
Right ventricle	28/8	15–30/0–8	75
Pulmonary artery	30/15	15–30/0–8	75
Left atrium (mean)	12	1–10	96
Left ventricle	165/12	100–140/3–12	97
Aorta	107/88	100–140/60–90	97

The most likely diagnosis is:

A aortic regurgitation
B aortic stenosis
C mitral regurgitation
D mitral stenosis
E ventricular septal defect

4.19 A 35-year-old woman was referred with an 8-month history of recurrent attacks of palpitations. There was no previous medical history and she did not drink or smoke.

On examination she was pain free. Her temperature was 36.9°C, pulse 66 regular and blood pressure 120/84. JVP was not elevated and heart sounds were normal. Chest, abdominal and neck examinations were normal. She had normal blood tests.

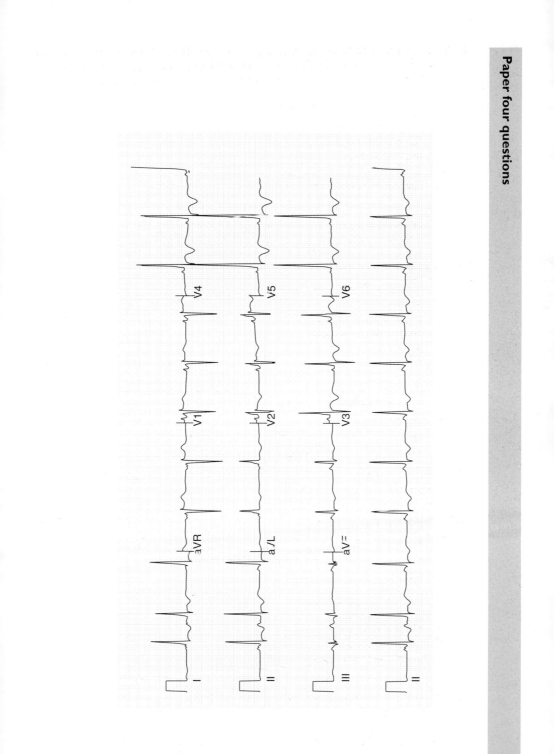

Her condition should be managed in the long term by:

A amiodarone
B digoxin
C implantable defibrillator
D permanent pacemaker
E radiofrequency ablation

4.20 A 21-year-old woman was admitted following a paracetamol overdose. She had been treated with N-acteylcysteine but after 4 days had failed to improve. She had become drowsier and it was difficult to understand her speech. She was jaundiced, had a coarse tremor and GCS score of 14/15. Her temperature was 37.3°C, pulse 92 regular and blood pressure 105/68, JVP +6 cm, heart sounds and chest clear. Her abdomen was soft and there was no ascites. Her urine output was 25 mL/hour.

Bloods	Hb	12.6	WCC	6.5
	Platelets	150	PT	42
	Na	134	K	4.0
	Urea	13.8	Creatinine	300
	Protein	64	Albumin	34
	Bilirubin	80	ALT	12,500
	ALP	340		

Arterial blood gases on air	pH	7.29	PCO_2	3.0
	PO_2	10.8		
	Bicarbonate	14.5	Base excess	−7.6

Which ONE of the following is NOT a determinant of whether this patient should be considered for liver transplantation?

A Acidosis in spite of fluid rehydration
B ALT
C Creatinine
D Encephalopathy grade
E Prothrombin time

4.21 A 22-year-old woman was referred with a non-pruritic, disfiguring rash on both forearms. She had no previous medical history and was on no medication (Figure 4.21). See plate section.

The treatment of choice for this patient is:

A coal tar soap
B hydrocortisone ointment
C observation and follow-up
D oral prednisolone
E topical clotrimazole

4.22 A 55-year-old man was referred with a 4-week history of weight loss, jaundice, dark urine, and pale stools but no abdominal pain. He had no previous medical history. He drank 2 units of alcohol per week and was a non-smoker. He was not on any medication and had not had any blood transfusions in the past. His last trip abroad was over 20 years ago.

On examination he was markedly jaundiced and looked thin. He was apyrexial, pulse 78 regular and blood pressure 120/70. His abdomen was soft and non-tender with 3 cm hepatomegaly below the costal margin.

Bloods	Hb	13.5	WCC	11.3
	Platelets	450	INR	1.1
	Na	135	K	4.2
	Urea	4.5	Creatinine	90
	Glucose	4.6	Bilirubin	96
	Albumin	30	Protein	60
	AST	60	ALP	300
	GGT	30		

Hepatitis A, B, C serology Negative

Abdominal ultrasound Mild hepatomegaly – normal echo texture

Normal common bile duct. Gallbladder empty with no stones seen

Dilated intrahepatic ducts

The most likely diagnosis is:

A autoimmune hepatitis
B carcinoma of head of pancreas
C lymphoma at porta hepatis
D primary biliary cirrhosis
E sclerosing cholangitis

4.23 It had been proposed that FOB could be used to screen for colorectal carcinoma. A trial using 1000 patients was carried out, 95 cases of carcinoma developed. The FOB detected 80 cases and 65 false-positives. The sensitivity of the FOB as a screening test is:

A 80/145
B 80/95
C 840/855
D 840/905
E 920/1000

4.24 A 50-year-old man in the intensive care unit had a 2-day history of jaundice. He was admitted following an emergency aortic aneurysm repair 2 weeks ago and had been slow to wean off ventilation. Five days ago he had developed cellulitis around the insertion of the CVP line in the right groin for which he had been started on intravenous antibiotics. He used to drink 2 units of alcohol most nights for 10 years. He had a previous medical history of hypercholesterolaemia but was not on any regular medication.

On examination he was alert and not being sedated. He had a tracheostomy and received mechanical ventilation. His temperature was 36.5°C, pulse 78 regular and blood pressure 145/92. His abdomen was soft and there was no organomegaly or distension. Rectal examination was normal. The abdominal wound site looked clean.

Bloods	Hb	12.5	MCV	84.6
	WCC	12.4	Platelets	180
	Albumin	28	Protein	54
	Bilirubin	135	ALT	50
	ALP	250	GGT	150
	INR	1.1		

Urinalysis Bilirubin 2+, no urobilinogen

The most likely cause of his deranged liver function is:

A ascending cholangitis
B autoimmune hepatitis
C decompensated liver disease secondary to alcoholic liver disease
D drug-induced cholestasis
E portal vein thrombosis

4.25 A 42-year-old man was referred with hepatomegaly and deranged liver function tests. He drunk 2 units of alcohol per day and was a heavy smoker. He had no risk factors for hepatitis. He had a normal appetite and stable weight.

On examination he was not jaundiced or pale. His pulse was 79 regular and blood pressure 140/89. His respiratory rate was 18 breaths/min and his chest was clear. He had 6 cm hepatomegaly but no other signs of chronic liver disease.

Bloods	Hb	13.4	WCC	4.5
	Platelets	110	INR	1.4
	Na	132	K	4.8
	Urea	3.9	Creatinine	80
	Albumin	33	Protein	70
	Bilirubin	30	ALT	85
	ALP	105	GGT	39
	Glucose	5.4		

Hepatitis A, B, C serology Negative

Liver biopsy (PAS-D)   Figure 4.25. See plate section.

The most likely diagnosis is:

A α_1-antitrypsin deficiency
B amyloidosis
C haemochromatosis
D hepatocellular carcinoma
E Wilson's disease

4.26 A 61-year-old man presented with difficulty in walking and weakness in his arms of recent onset. He had no visual or speech problems. His bladder and bowels were normal.

On examination there was generalised weakness and wasting of the muscles of the hands, arms and shoulders and with fasciculation. There was reduced tone and upper limb reflexes were decreased. In the lower limbs there was weakness of the lower limb muscles with increased tone and reflexes. Plantar responses were extensor. Pinprick, light touch, vibration sense and proprioception were normal throughout. His gait was 'scissors-like'.

The most likely diagnosis is:

A cervical myelopathy
B Charcot–Marie–Tooth disease
C motor neurone disease
D poliomyelitis
E syringomyelia

4.27 A 55-year-old man was admitted with shortness of breath and abdominal pain. He had suffered from osteoarthritis and took diclofenac. He was a heavy smoker but did not drink alcohol.

Arterial blood gases on air	pH	7.11	PCO_2	6.5
	PO_2	10.2	Bicarbonate	12
	Base excess	−14		

These blood gases show:

    A metabolic acidosis and respiratory alkalosis with no respiratory failure
    B mixed metabolic and respiratory acidosis with no respiratory failure
    C mixed metabolic and respiratory acidosis with respiratory failure
    D respiratory acidosis and metabolic alkalosis with no respiratory failure
    E respiratory acidosis with no respiratory failure

4.28 A 30-year-old Philippino women was referred with a 2-month history of fever, arthralgia affecting shoulders and neck and some weight loss. She also complained of dizziness and some leg and chest pain that occurred with exercise. She had no previous medical history and was not on any medication. She did not smoke or drink alcohol.

On examination she looked well. Her temperature was 37.4°C, her radial pulses were difficult to feel but at the apex her heart rate was 88 regular and blood pressure 148/90. Her JVP was not elevated and both heart sounds were normal. She had bilateral carotid bruits. Respiratory and abdominal examination was normal. Her legs looked normal but she experienced pain on raising them 35° from the horizontal. She had no focal neurological deficit.

Bloods	Hb	12.3	WCC	4.8
	Platelets	259	Na	140
	K	4.1	Urea	5.8
	Creatinine	89	Protein	68
	Albumin	39	Bilirubin	10
	ALT	25	ALP	73
	ESR	58	CRP	38
	PT	12	APTT	25

Rheumatoid factor	Negative
Antinuclear antibody	Negative
Chest X-ray	Normal
ECG	No ischaemic changes

The most likely diagnosis is:

    A antiphospholipid syndrome
    B Kawasaki's disease
    C polyarteritis nodosa
    D Takayasu's arteritis
    E type A dissection of ascending aorta

4.29 This 55-year-old man was admitted with recent abdominal pain, weight loss, jaundice and ascites. He did not drink alcohol.

On examination he was cachectic and mildly jaundiced. Abdomen was tender with gross ascites. An ascitic tap was performed; the fluid aspirated is shown (Figure 4.29). See plate section.

The most likely diagnosis is:

A Budd–Chiari syndrome
B nephrotic syndrome
C acute pancreatitis
D constrictive pericarditis
E lymphoma

4.30 A 43-year-old woman had pain in both hands. She was undergoing renal dialysis (Figure 4.30). See plate section.

The most likely cause for the pain is:

A gout
B hyperparathyroidism
C Paget's disease
D rheumatoid arthritis
E sarcoidosis

4.31 A 48-year-old Armenian refugee was admitted with shortness of breath and haemoptysis. No previous history was available.

On examination he was unwell and breathless. His temperature was 38.0°C, pulse 90 regular and blood pressure 120/60. His respiratory rate was 30 breaths/min and there were bilateral crackles on auscultation (Figure 4.31). See plate section.

Apart from oxygen, the most appropriate treatment for this patient is:

A aciclovir
B cefuroxime and clarithromycin
C furosemide (frusemide)
D hydrocortisone
E rifampicin, isoniazid, pyrazinamide and ethambutol

4.32 A 61-year-old man was referred with worsening shortness of breath on exertion over the past 5 months with associated attacks of central chest pain that also occurred at rest. He could walk about 200 metres before being stopped by dyspnoea. He slept with three pillows but sometimes had breathlessness at night. He did not smoke. He had had rheumatic fever as a child.

On examination he was breathless at rest. His pulse was 74 regular and blood pressure 120/90. His JVP was not elevated and his carotid pulse was difficult to palpate. There was a loud ejection systolic murmur that radiated to both carotids. There were bilateral crackles at both bases.

Which one of the following statements concerning management of his condition is correct?

A The louder the murmur the more severe the condition
B An ACE inhibitor is the best treatment option
C A bioprosthetic rather than mechanical valve replacement would give longer life-expectancy
D Valve replacement should be performed if the surface area of the valve is less than $0.8\,cm^2$
E Balloon valvuloplasty is the treatment of choice

4.33 A 73-year-old man was visiting his wife in hospital when he collapsed. A cardiac monitor showed the following trace. There was no palpable pulse.

The next step in the immediate management of this patient would be:

A adrenaline (epinephrine) 1 mg intravenously
B defibrillate 200 J
C lidocaine (lignocaine) 100 mg intravenously
D precordial thump
E start cardiopulmonary chest compressions

4.34 A 19-year-old student complained of a painless rash on his penis and some dysuria (Figure 4.39). See plate section.

The rash shows:

A condyloma accuminata
B chancroid
C primary chancre
D circinate balanitis
E herpes genitalis

4.35 A 35-year-old woman was referred with a 10-week history of galactor-rhoea and loss of menstrual periods. She also complained of loss of libido and headaches. She was not on any medication.

On examination there was no focal neurological defect. Breast examination was normal.

Bloods	Na	140	K	4.1
	Urea	5.2	Creatinine	78
	TSH	4	Free T$_4$	20
	Prolactin	1450		

Urine β-HCG Negative

MRI pituitary Microadenoma

The most appropriate treatment for this patient is:

A amitriptyline
B bromocriptine
C cimetidine
D metoclopramide
E oestrogen

4.36 A 15-year-old girl was admitted with abdominal pain and bloody diarrhoea. She opened her bowels up to 10 times a day, passing blood and mucus. A provisional diagnosis of inflammatory bowel disease was made and the consultant in charge of her care suggested a colonoscopy would help with the diagnosis. The benefits and risks with colonoscopy were explained to the patient who appeared to understand what the procedure involved. She agreed to have the procedure but unfortunately her mother objected to the test being performed and refused to allow it.

The correct management plan for this patient would be to:

A explore other options of investigating this patient's bowel condition
B obtain a court order to perform the procedure
C postpone the procedure until the mother changes her mind
D proceed with the colonoscopy, as the patient has given informed consent
E proceed with the colonoscopy, as the consultant in charge of the patient's care can take full responsibility for inpatient care because she is aged under 16

4.37 A 35-year-old woman was admitted with abdominal pain and increasing abdominal distension over the past 3 weeks. She had no relevant previous medical history. She did not drink or smoke. She was not pregnant and was on the oral contraceptive pill. She was on no other medication.

On examination she looked ill but was alert and orientated. She was apyrexial and mildly icteric. Her pulse was 100 regular and blood pressure 95/60. Cardiovascular and respiratory examinations were normal. She had gross ascites and generalised abdominal tenderness. Rectal examination was normal.

Bloods	Hb	12.5	WCC	10.5
	Platelets	85	INR	1.4
	Na	135	K	4.5
	Urea	8.5	Creatinine	200
	Albumin	24	Protein	56
	Bilirubin	40	ALT	1200
	ALP	140	GGT	100
	Amylase	58		

Hepatitis A, B, C serology Negative

Paracetamol Not detected

Salicylate Not detected

Chest X-ray Normal

Abdominal X-ray No evidence of obstruction

Abdominal ultrasound
Gross ascites
Hepatomegaly with an enlarged caudate lobe
Splenomegaly
Portal vein and inferior vena cava patent

The most likely diagnosis is:

    A autoimmune hepatitis
    B Budd–Chiari syndrome
    C ecstasy overdose
    D metastatic disease
    E portal vein thrombosis

4.38 A 42-year-old man presented with a 5-week history of severe pain and paresthesiae in his back radiating down his leg. It came on gradually and he found walking difficult. The right side was worse than the left. There were no symptoms in his arms or face. He had no bowel or bladder problems. He had a previous medical history of diabetes mellitus for which he was on insulin. He had no eye or renal complications.

On examination he had weakness of his plantar flexors, peroneus longus, extensor digitorum brevis and hamstrings. Tone was normal but power was reduced. Knee jerk was intact but ankle reflex was absent; plantar responses were flexor. There was decreased sensation to light touch and pinprick over the lateral border of the foot.

His neurological abnormalities are due to:

A myelopathy
B myopathy
C peripheral neuropathy
D radiculopathy
E subcortical lesion

4.39 A 47-year-old smoker was referred with haemoptysis. Chest X-ray revealed a left hilar lesion. At bronchoscopy an endobronchial tumour was found, which histology confirmed as squamous cell carcinoma. Liver ultrasound showed no evidence of metastases.

Surgical resection of the tumour might still be possible in the presence of:

A dysphagia
B elevated left hemidiaphragm on chest x-ray
C hypercalcaemia
D hoarse voice
E predicted postoperative FEV_1 of 0.7 L

4.40 A 28-year-old male was referred with pain and stiffness in his right knee for about 1 week. Since then that pain had resolved, but now his hands and wrists were painful. He had a rash on his penis and complained of dysuria and creamy discharge. He was heterosexual but had multiple sexual partners.

On examination his temperature was 37.5°C, pulse 88 regular and blood pressure 130/74. Respiratory and abdominal systems were normal. The right knee joint looked normal. Both wrists and metacarpo-phalangeal joints were mildly inflamed with some inflammation and tenderness of the tendon sheaths. There was a small, painless ulcer on his penis and small, tender vesicles on the back of the hands and wrists.

Bloods				
Hb	12.0	WCC	11.8
Platelets	480	Neutrophils	7.5
Na	137	K	4.2
Urea	5.7	Creatinine	89
Protein	70	Albumin	40
Bilirubin	10	ALT	25
ALP	70	ESR	34
CRP	40		

Synovial fluid Slightly turbid appearance

WCC	40,000	Neutrophils	60%
No growth		Protein	35

Urine culture No growth

Blood cultures Awaited

The most likely diagnosis is:

A ankylosing spondylitis
B Behçet's syndrome
C gonococcal arthritis
D primary syphilis
E Reiter's syndrome

4.41 A 16-year-old girl presented with sudden onset cough and shortness of breath. She suffered from asthma that was well controlled. She had no calf swelling. There was no significant family history and she had not been abroad recently.

On examination she was in some distress using her accessory muscles of respiration. Temperature was 36.5°C, pulse 110 regular and blood pressure 100/60. Her respiratory rate was 30 breaths/min but no wheeze was heard (Figure 4.41). See plate section.

| **Arterial blood** | pH | 7.34 | PCO$_2$ | 3.6 |
| **gases on air** | PO$_2$ | 9.4 | | |

The reason for her breathlessness is:

A hysterical hyperventilation
B inhaled foreign body
C inspissated mucus plug blocking small airways
D pneumothorax
E pulmonary embolism

4.42 A 49-year-old man presented with progressive shortness of breath and dysphagia (Figure 4.42). See plate section.

The chest X-ray findings would be most consistent with:

A Hodgkin's lymphoma
B retrosternal goitre
C teratoma
D thoracic aortic aneurysm
E thymoma

4.43 A 13-year-old boy was referred by social services because of bruises and scars on his body. Other than generalised bruising, he had epicanthal folds and a flat nasal bridge (Figure 4.43). See plate section.

The most likely diagnosis is:

A Ehlers–Danlos syndrome
B Marfan's syndrome
C Noonan's syndrome
D osteogenesis imperfecta
E pseudoxanthoma elasticum

4.44 A 57-year-old woman was referred because of 4-month history of shortness of breath and peripheral oedema. She denied chest pain or palpitations. Her exercise tolerance was reduced to approximately 100 metres and she now required three pillows to prevent breathlessness at night. She had a longstanding history of rheumatoid arthritis affecting her wrists and elbows, which was not active and she was taking methotrexate.

On examination she had peripheral oedema up to the sacrum. Her pulse was 88 regular and blood pressure 110/90. Her JVP was elevated +8 cm and there were no murmurs but she did have third and fourth heart sounds. Her chest was clear. There was hepatomegaly and arthritic deformities of both hands and wrists with nodules at her elbows.

Bloods				
	Hb	12.8	WCC	8.5
	Platelets	245	INR	1.1
	Na	135	K	4.3
	Urea	6.6	Creatinine	110
	Albumin	33	Protein	70
	Bilirubin	14	ALT	45
	ALP	70		

Chest X-ray   Normal heart size

No pulmonary oedema

ECG   T wave inversion in I, aVL, V_{4-6}

The most likely diagnosis is:

  A dilated cardiomyopathy
  B drug-induced myocarditis
  C hypertrophic obstructive cardiomyopathy
  D Libman–Sacks endocarditis
  E restrictive cardiomyopathy

4.45 A 25-year-old man with a history of Crohn's disease was referred with abdominal pain. There was no nausea or vomiting, his appetite was normal and he had not lost weight. He opened his bowels once a day and his stools were solid with some mucus but no blood. He was only on mesalazine tablets. He had a colonoscopy a year ago when Crohn's disease was diagnosed, which showed quiescent disease up to the caecum.

On examination he was apyrexial. There was generalised abdominal tenderness but no masses and rectal examination was normal.

The next most appropriate investigation would be:

    A barium enema
    B CT abdomen
    C radiolabelled white cell scan
    D repeat colonoscopy
    E small bowel follow-through

4.46 A 16-year-old girl was referred because of a 2-month history of seizures. They began with her seeing flashing lights and continued with jerking of the left upper limb for up to 5 minutes. Occasionally she had bitten her tongue but had never lost control of her bowels or bladder. She did not lose consciousness when fitting and had no postseizure amnesia. She had no previous medical history; she was not on any medication and there was no family history of epilepsy.

    On examination she looked well and there was no abnormalities found on physical examination.

Full blood count   Normal

Urea and electrolytes Normal

The most likely diagnosis is:

    A absence seizures
    B complex partial siezures
    C myoclonic seizures
    D simple partial seizures
    E tonic clonic seizures

4.47 A breathless 45-year-old man was referred for lung function tests:

	Absolute	Predicted (%)
FEV_1	1.2	33
FVC	2.6	55
TLC	5.5	112
DLCO	8.3	38
KCO	1.5	42

The results would be most consistent with:

    A atrial septal defect with left to right shunt
    B emphysema
    C extrinsic allergic alveolitis
    D pulmonary embolus
    E sarcoidosis

4.48 A 26-year-old man was referred because of progressively worsening pain in his spine, hips and knees over the past 4 months. He also complained of skin darkening, especially his ears. In addition to this, his urine darkened markedly if it was allowed to stand. His father also suffered a similar problem.

On examination his skin was hyperpigmented and his ears were blue-black in colour. His pulse was 92 regular and blood pressure 110/82. His JVP was not elevated but there was an ejection systolic murmur. His chest was clear. There was loss of the lumbar lordosis and he had difficulty stooping forward. The knee joints were swollen and inflamed. There was no neurological deficit.

Lumbosacral X-ray   Calcification of the intervertebral discs

Narrowing of the intervertebral spaces

The most likely diagnosis is:

A alkaptonuria
B ankylosing spondylitis
C homocystinuria
D maple syrup urine disease
E relapsing polychondritis

4.49 A 40-year-old man was admitted with worsening shortness of breath and cough productive of thick yellow sputum. This had been progressing over 2 years and it was his fourth admission this year. He was a smoker until he stopped last year.

On examination he was breathless and cyanosed. His temperature was 37.2°C, pulse 110 regular and blood pressure 120/78. His respiratory rate was 30 breaths/min and there were bilateral crackles in his lungs (Figure 4.49). See plate section.

The condition that would be **LEAST** likely to have caused his chest X-ray appearances is:

A aspergillosis
B childhood pertussis infection
C chronic obstructive pulmonary disease
D cystic fibrosis
E tuberculosis

4.50 A 68-year-old man complained of a lump that had been growing on the top of his scalp for the past 2 months (Figure 4.50). See plate section.

Which **ONE** of the following is **LEAST** likely to be the cause of the scalp lesion?

A arsenic exposure
B burn scars
C immunosuppressant treatment postrenal transplant
D pigmented naevi
E PUVA (psoralen + ultraviolet A light) treatment

4.51 A 22-year-old patient was referred with infertility. He had been married for 1 year but had so far failed to make his wife pregnant. He was very embarrassed, describing that he did have breasts and that his genitalia were not very big. He had no previous medical history and did not smoke or drink alcohol.

On examination he was somewhat short but had a normal appearance. He was clinically euthyroid. There was gynaecomastia and both testes were present, albeit very small.

Bloods	Testosterone	5.5	(normal: 10–29 nmol/L)
	FSH	40	(normal: 1–7 U/L)
	LH	28	(normal: 1–6 U/L)

Sperm count Azoospermia

The most likely karyotype of this patient is:

A 45,XO
B 46,XO
C 46,XY
D 47,XXY
E 47,XYY

4.52 A 35-year-old man was found to have a colonic tumour on colonoscopy. His father had developed carcinoma of the rectum aged 55 and his uncle had died from colonic carcinoma aged 60. He had a total colectomy and made an uneventful recovery.

The syndrome this patient is likely to have is:

A familial adenomatous polyposis
B Gardner's syndrome
C hereditary non-polyposis colorectal cancer
D juvenile polyposis
E Peutz–Jeghers syndrome

4.53 A 35-year-old woman presented with worsening headaches and blurred vision. Over the past 3 months she had also noticed a 4 kg weight loss and an itchy rash on her legs. Her only previous medical history was of peptic ulcer disease that was diagnosed last year but responded to high dose proton pump inhibitors.

On examination she looked cachexic. There was a widespread erythematous rash on both lower limbs. There was no jaundice or lymphadenopathy. Epigastric tenderness was the only finding on examination of the abdomen. On testing the visual fields she had bitemporal hemianopia.

Bloods
Calcium	2.70	Phosphate	0.55
Albumin	32	Glucose	13.4
PTH	6.9	Prolactin	1000

The most likely diagnosis is:

A APS 1
B APS 2
C MEN 1 syndrome
D MEN 2A syndrome
E MEN 2B syndrome

4.54 A 70-year-old woman admitted with acute abdominal pain. She had had similar symptoms with irregular bowel habit on and off for the past 3 months. This time the pain was very severe and she had passed some fresh blood per rectum. She had no previous medical history and was not on any medication.

On examination she had a temperature of 38.0°C, pulse 95 regular and blood pressure 110/60. There was tenderness in the left iliac fossa, no organomegaly and rectal examination revealed some blood but no masses.

Bloods
Hb	10.5	WCC	13.5
Neutrophils	11.7	Platelets	345
Na	140	K	4.5
Urea	7.8	Creatinine	96
Albumin	30	Protein	60
Bilirubin	10	ALT	20
ALP	70	GGT	35
Amylase	50	CRP	120
ESR	55		

Chest X-ray Normal

Abdominal X-ray No evidence of obstruction

The most likely diagnosis is:

A acute diverticulitis
B Crohn's disease
C ischaemic colitis
D ovarian carcinoma
E pseudomembranous colitis

4.55 A 70-year-old woman was brought in drowsy and confused. Her daughter said that she had been off her food and had vomited several times that day.

She had decreased skin turgor and a furred tongue. Her temperature was 38.2°C. Pulse was 105 regular, blood pressure 100/55 and her JVP was not elevated. Heart sounds and chest were normal. Respiratory rate was 16 breaths per minute. There was vague lower abdominal tenderness. She was unable to walk independently.

Bloods	Hb	12.5	WCC	13.4
	Platelets	200	Na	158
	K	4.0	Urea	19.0
	Creatinine	184	Glucose	58
Blood gases on air	pH	7.37	PCO_2	4.6
	PO_2	10.5	Bicarbonate	28

Urine osmolality 300 mosmol/kg

Urinanalysis Protein 2+, glucose 3+, ketones 1+

Which **ONE** of the following statements concerning this patient's management is **FALSE**?

A Her blood glucose should be brought down as quickly as possible
B If she becomes more drowsy she should have an nasogastric tube inserted
C She may not need to be put on any long-term antidiabetic medication
D She should be given 0.45% saline
E She should be given prophylactic heparin

4.56 A 49-year-old man was referred with left loin pain and haematuria. He had a long history of renal stones. He had no other medical problems and was on no medication.

On examination his temperature was 36.5°C, pulse 88 regular and blood pressure 148/92. There was tenderness in the left loin region but no organomegaly and rectal examination was normal.

Bloods	Hb	10.9	MCV	96.4
	WCC	8.6	Platelets	200
	Na	138	K	3.1
	Urea	18.3	Creatinine	220
	Protein	68	Albumin	38
	Bicarbonate	10	Chloride	114
	Calcium	2.42	Phosphate	0.98
	Renin (upright)	3.4		
	Aldosterone (upright)	420		

Urinanalysis pH 6.4, protein 2+, blood 1+, white cells 1+

Abdominal X-ray Speckled calcification of both kidneys

The most likely diagnosis is:

A Bartter's syndrome
B Conn's syndrome
C renal tubular acidosis I
D renal tubular acidosis II
E renal tubular acidosis IV

4.57 A 27-year-old man presented with pyrexia for the past 7 days. He had just returned back from a holiday in the Gambia (Figure 4.57). See plate section.

The organism seen in the film is:

A *Leishmania donovani*
B *Loa loa*
C *Plasmodium falciparum*
D *Schistosoma haematobium*
E *Trypanosoma brucei gambiense*

4.58 A 28-year-old woman was referred with jaundice, neck stiffness and headache. She also complained of red, gritty eyes. Her symptoms had started 7 days ago as a flu-like illness and had got progressively worse. She had just returned from a camping holiday in the USA in the Grand Canyon. There was no previous medical history and she was not on any medication. She did not drink alcohol or smoke.

On examination she was jaundiced and had bilateral conjunctivitis. Her temperature was 38.2°C, pulse 100 regular and blood pressure 120/90. Her JVP was not elevated and heart sounds were normal. Chest was clear. There was some right upper quadrant tenderness but no organomegaly. She was not encephalopathic, Kernig's sign was positive but the rest of the neurological examination was normal. There was no skin rash.

Bloods				
Hb	11.9		MCV	93.0
WCC	12.3		Neutrophils	10.1
Lymphocytes	1.9		Eosinophils	0.3
Platelets	259		Na	138
K	4.4		Urea	5.5
Creatinine	80		Protein	70
Albumin	35		Bilirubin	65
ALT	145		ALP	135
CRP	189			

Chest X-ray Normal

The most likely diagnosis is:

A hepatitis A
B histoplasmosis
C leptospirosis
D Lyme disease
E Rocky Mountain spotted fever

4.59 A 45-year-old woman was referred with widespread cervical and inguinal lymphadenopathy that was diagnosed as Hodgkin's lymphoma. She felt otherwise well. Physical examination was normal apart from the lymphadenopathy.

Which **ONE** of the following is associated with a **BETTER** prognosis.

A lymphocyte-predominant disease
B mediastinal disease
C night sweats
D splenic involvement
E subdiaphragmatic disease

4.60 A 13-year-old boy was referred because of painless haematuria. He had no cough or shortness of breath. Sensorineural deafness had been diagnosed at the age of 5. His mother also had renal impairment. He was not on any medication.

On examination his pulse was 80 regular and blood pressure 90/50. Abdominal examination was normal.

Bloods	Hb	12.4	WCC	4.5
	Platelets	250	Na	138
	K	4.0	Urea	4.8
	Creatinine	79	Protein	70
	Albumin	39	Calcium	2.33
	Glucose	4.5		

Urinanalysis pH 6.4, blood 2+

Retrograde pyelography Normal

Cystoscopy Normal

The most likely diagnosis is:

A Alport's syndrome
B autosomal dominant polycystic kidney disease
C Fabry's disease
D juvenile nephronophthisis
E thin basement membrane nephritis

Paper 4

Answers

4.1 **B**** This patient has 'lone atrial fibrillation'. He has no other medical conditions so he would be considered a low risk for cerebrovascular disease. From the Stroke Prevention in Atrial Fibrillation study, patients under 65 with lone atrial fibrillation would benefit from aspirin, not warfarin.

Stroke Prevention in Atrial Fibrillation II Study. Warfarin versus aspirin for prevention of thromboembolism in atrial fibrillation. (1994) *Lancet* **343(8899):**687–91.

4.2 **D***** The PR interval is prolonged and there are two P waves for each QRS complex. This is fixed 2:1 atrioventricular block.

4.3 **B***** This patient has bradycardia, hypotension and dilated pupils suggestive of a beta-blocker overdose. Tricyclic antidepressant overdose would typically cause a tachyarrythmia. Digoxin would be expected to cause heart block but should not cause mydriasis. Codeine phosphate, as an opiate would be expected to cause constricted pupils.

4.4 **A**** Impetigo is a superficial skin infection caused by staphylococci and streptococci. It starts with small, red macules that give way to small, fluid-filled vesicles. On top of these form honey-yellow crusting exudates, which may coalesce and enlarge. There may be associated pyrexia and painful lymphadenopathy.

4.5 **A**** The symptoms of cough, weight loss and abdominal pain, which he may have contracted abroad, are suggestive of tuberculosis. There is hyponatraemia, hyperkalaemia and hypoglycaemia. Hyponatraemia is possibly due to the adrenal glands failing to produce aldosterone and the hyperkalaemia is due to the relative deficiency of aldosterone, which helps excrete potassium. Postural hypotension is associated with Addison's disease and is due to relative hypovolaemia and hyponatraemia.

4.6 **A**** Of all the proposals, the only one that would be appropriate as an RCT would be investigating whether atenolol could prevent recurrence of stroke. RCTs are primarily used to test the efficacy of a treatment or intervention and not for diagnosis, determining causality or predicting prognosis.

4.7 **B***** This patient has all the features of Charcot's triad (fever, abdominal pain and jaundice) and so cholangitis is the diagnosis until proven otherwise. Ultrasound should always be performed in the jaundiced patient to see if there is dilatation of the common bile duct and if there are residual stones. Blood cultures would identify the organism and hence confirm the diagnosis. *E. coli, Enterococcus* and *Pseudomonas* spp are the most likely organisms. ERCP may be necessary to remove a stone in the common bile duct that is acting as the source of infection; but as no mention of an ultrasound report, ERCP should not be first line investigation and may not give the diagnosis. The patient has a temperature of >39°C, so taking blood cultures is mandatory.

4.8 **C**** To diagnose PRV, secondary causes of erythrocytosis need to be excluded. These include Gaisböck's syndrome where there is polycythaemia secondary to hypoxia and renal tumours With PRV, there is usually leukocytosis and increased neutrophil alkaline phosphatase score in the absence of infection. There may be an iron deficiency anaemia but there is increased vitamin B_{12} due to increased binding protein transcobalamin I; serum folate is normal. In PRV the serum erythropoietin level would be low, indicating an autonomous proliferative disorder.

4.9 **A**** The slide shows *Aspergillus fumigatus* with the characteristic septated hyphae. The chest X-ray shows two lesions on the right side of the chest, which could represent an aspergilloma. This represents the growth within previously damaged lung tissue of *A. fumigatus*.

4.10 **E**** Treatment of chronic hepatitis C is contemplated in patients who are symptomatic and have deranged liver function tests. The aim of treatment is to try and prevent cirrhosis in patients with actively replicating virus. The latter is suggested by a positive HCV PCR RNA. Next, the genotype of the virus needs to be identified, as this will determine the duration of treatment. There are six genotypes, of which genotype 1 is the most resistant to treatment. With all genotypes, treatment is given for 6 months with ribavirin and α-interferon. Only patients with genotype 1 who have shown clinical improvement with treatment are given a further 6 months of antiviral treatment. Azathioprine and prednisolone are used to treat autoimmune hepatitis; lamivudine is used to treat hepatitis B.

4.11 **B***** This woman has myasthenia gravis with the characteristic fatigability of neuromuscular junction disease. Myasthenia gravis is an autoimmune disease involving antibodies targeted against the acetylcholine receptors of the neuromuscular junction. It can affect limb muscles as well as the ocular and bulbar muscles. It does not affect the heart and so there are no cardiac abnormalities, but the shortness of breath is due to respiratory muscle involvement. Eaton–Lambert syndrome is also a disorder of neuromuscular transmission but is due to antibodies targeting the presynaptic voltage-gated calcium channels. Unlike myasthenia gravis, muscle strength may improve for a short while after exercise. Also, this condition tends to affect the proximal limb muscles, not involve the bulbar muscles and can be associated with hyporeflexia. Over 60% of cases are associated with small cell carcinoma of the lung. A peripheral neuropathy could not account for all these symptoms.

4.12 C** The picture shows a segment of a white fluffy area radiating out from the disc. The rest of the disc looks normal. These areas are characteristic of myelinated fibres and do not affect vision.

4.13 A** This patient has a right lobar pneumonia, most probably due to *Streptococcus pneumoniae* acquired in the community. The vast majority of these are still sensitive to penicillin and so amoxicillin would be a sensible choice. There is nothing in the history to suggest that this is tuberculosis or legionnaire's disease.

British Thoracic Society (2001) Guidelines for the management of community acquired pneumonia in adults. *Thorax* **56**(supplement IV).

4.14 E*** The only fully consistent diagnosis is SLE with at least four of the diagnostic criteria: discoid rash, non-erosive arthritis, ANA-positive, positive anti-SM antibodies, evidence of haematological disorder (leukopenia, thrombocytopenia and normocytic anaemia), evidence of renal disorder and possible serositis. Rheumatoid arthritis and mixed connective tissue disease are not associated with positive anti-SM antibodies. Unlike other arthritides, SLE often has a persistently high ESR and a normal CRP. Low C3 and C4 can be associated with SLE-induced nephritis. Anti-Ro and Anti-La antibodies may be positive in SLE patients but these are usually the patients with Sjögren's overlap. Churg–Strauss syndrome can involve lungs and kidneys but there is little associated arthritis and c-ANCA is positive.

4.15 D*** This patient has a puffy, thickened myxoedematous face with dry, pale skin and a slight malar flush.

4.16 A** The CT shows a low density area in the middle cerebral artery territory extending to the cortex, with some mass effect in the left frontoparietal region. This is an acute infarct because the lesion appears hypodense/low attenuation (dark).

4.17 C** This barium swallow shows a long stricture with irregular shouldering. This is most likely to be an oesophageal neoplasm.

4.18 B*** Normally with cardiac catheterisation there should not be large pressure differences as blood crosses between chambers. In this case there is a large pressure drop between the left ventricle and the aorta. This would suggest a stenotic lesion. If there were aortic regurgitation, there would be a large pulse pressure in the aorta.

4.19 E** This patient has Wolff–Parkinson–White syndrome with a short PR interval and the slurring upstroke of the delta wave. The treatment of choice is radiofrequency ablation of the accessory pathway.

4.20 B** This patient has developed hyperacute liver failure, as she has developed encephalopathy within 7 days of jaundice. The King's College transplant criteria for paracetamol-induced liver failure include: (1) pH<7.3 following rehydration and at greater than 24 hours after overdose; (2) grade III/IV encephalopathy; (3) creatinine >300; (4) PT >100. Not all the criteria have to be met but the above should occur on the same day. It is for this reason that, unless a patient is bleeding, fresh frozen plasma should **NOT** be given to correct the coagulopathy.

4.21 C*** This patient has dermatitis artefacta. The lesions are multiple, bear no resemblance to any dermatological disease and are in easy reach of the patient's hands, and physical discomfort is minimal. She needs psychiatric assessment.

4.22 C*** A man presents with progressive, painless obstructive jaundice and weight loss, as confirmed by dark urine, pale stools and cholestatic liver function tests. The ultrasound report shows dilated intrahepatic ducts in the absence of common bile duct dilatation; this suggests a stricture/obstruction more proximal in the biliary tree. The only two responses compatible with that diagnosis are obstruction at the porta hepatis or sclerosing cholangitis. This is less likely to be primary sclerosing cholangitis because there is no previous medical history, particularly no history of inflammatory bowel disease. The cachexia would be in keeping with underlying malignancy, although primary sclerosing cholangitis can be associated with cholangiocarcinoma.

4.23 B*** The sensitivity is the proportion of patients who have the condition that are detected by the test.

	Colon cancer +	Colon cancer –	
FOB +	80 (a)	65 (b)	145
FOB –	15 (c)	840 (d)	855
	95	905	1000

Sensitivity = a/a + c = 80/95 = 0.84

4.24 D** This is most likely to be cholestasis induced by flucloxacillin started for his cellulitis. Decompensated liver disease can occur especially after major operations but there is nothing to suggest he had this in the first place. Gallstones, likewise, may cause cholangitis but he is not pyrexial and does not complain of abdominal pain. The low globulin and raised ALP and GGT go against a picture of autoimmune hepatitis.

4.25 A* This slide shows periportal hepatocytes; the portal venule is to the extreme left-hand side. The purple globules are the α_1-antitrypsin, which accumulates and cannot be exported. PAS-D is the stain used to diagnose α_1-antitrypsin deficiency.

4.26 C* Motor neurone disease is a progressive disease of upper and lower motor neurones and can be classified as amyotrophic lateral sclerosis, progressive multiple atrophy and progressive bulbar palsy. There are no sensory signs, or evidence of cerebellar, extrapyramidal or dementia disease. With progressive bulbar palsy patients may present with nasal speech, wasted fasciculating tongue and palatal paralysis. Cervical myelopathy would need to be excluded but one would expect some sensory involvement. Polio may resemble progressive muscular atrophy but exclusively affects the lower motor neurone. Sensory abnormalities would be expected in syringomyelia and HSMN.

4.27 B This patient has respiratory acidosis, as evidenced by a low pH and raised PCO_2. There is also a low bicarbonate and a negative base excess, suggesting a metabolic acidosis as well. The PO_2 is above 8 and so there is no evidence of respiratory failure. These results would be consistent with chronic obstructive airways disease and intra-abdominal perforation. For an explanation of arterial blood gas interpretation, see **1.30**.

4.28 D Takayasu's arteritis is a large vessel vasculitis and is associated with bruits, claudication, decreased pulses, hypertension, arthralgias and neurological symptoms. There are no specific tests but it is more common in young Asian women, although all racial groups are affected. Antiphospholipid syndrome would be unlikely given her lack of rash, normal platelet count, normal APTT and negative ANA.

4.29 E The ascitic tap reveals chylous ascites, which is associated with obstruction of the thoracic duct and other major lymphatics. Acute pancreatitis doesn't usually result in ascites but when it does it may be haemorrhagic. The other causes usually produce straw-coloured ascites.

4.30 B The X-ray shows subperiosteal bone resorption, bony erosions and some soft tissue and arterial calcification. These are all the hallmarks of hyperparathyroidism.

4.31 E* This refugee's chest X-ray and his history of haemoptysis suggest that he has miliary tuberculosis. He should be isolated while infectious and started on 'quadruple therapy'.

4.32 D This patient has signs of aortic stenosis. The intensity of the murmur is related more to the cardiac output than the severity of his condition. The decision to replace the valve depends on whether the patient is symptomatic: syncope, angina or heart failure; has an aortic valve gradient greater than 50 mmHg; or the valve has a surface area less than 0.8 cm^2 (normal area is 2.5–3.0 cm^2). There is no difference in prognosis between bioprosthetic valves and mechanical valves, even though the former would avoid the need for life-long anticoagulation. Aortic valves are easy to replace; mitral valves are more likely to be repaired because of the difficulty in cutting the chordae tendinae in replacing the valve.

4.33 E** The cardiac monitor shows asystole. According to the universal treatment algorithm for non-VT/VF, cardiopulmonary resuscitation should be attempted. In this case chest compressions followed by atropine 3 mg intravenously and then 1 mg adrenaline (epinephrine) after one 3-minute cycle of chest compressions.

4.34 B* Circinate balanitis is characterised by small flesh-red erosions, with well-defined margins, which may coalesce. They may cause itching or burning but are often painless. Circinate balanitis and keratoderma blennorrhagicum are characteristic of Reiter's disease. Herpes simplex infection is associated with painful small ulcers that become vesicles which may burst to leave crusting erosions. Chancres are associated with primary syphilis and usually present as painless, indurated ulcers. Chancroid is a disease caused by *Haemophilus ducreyi* and often presents as one or more painful ulcers with a raised and undermined margin. There may also be associated lymphadenopathy.

4.35 B** This patient has increased prolactin secretion due to a prolactinoma. To diagnose prolactinoma, thyroid and renal disease have to be excluded as well as drug causes. The main regulatory factor in the release of prolactin is tonic inhibition of dopamine secretion by the hypothalamus. MRI pituitary would show the difference between a (non-functioning) macroadenoma and a microadenoma (i.e. differentiate between a tumour invading the pituitary stalk and a prolactin-secreting tumour). The treatment of a prolactinoma involves using bromocriptine, a dopamine agonist, with surgery reserved for tumours that do not respond to medical treatment or non-functioning macroadenomas. The other drugs listed can cause high prolactin levels.

4.36 D** According to the General Medical Council's guidelines on consent, if a child is under age 16 he or she may give consent if the child is deemed to have the capacity to understand what the procedure involves and does not require the parent's permission. Where a competent child refuses treatment, a person with parental responsibility or a court may authorise treatment or investigation if it is in the child's best interest.

4.37 B** The most likely diagnosis is Budd–Chiari sydrome, which is due to thrombosis of the three hepatic veins (right, middle and left). The caudate lobe of the liver drains directly into the inferior vena cava; if a block occurs to the hepatic veins then there is compensatory hypertrophy of the caudate lobe, making it look enlarged on ultrasound or CT. There are a number of causes of Budd–Chiari sydrome: abdominal trauma; myeloproliferative disease; hepatocellular carcinoma; paroxysmal nocturnal haemoglobinuria; certain tumours like those of the adrenal, pancreas and kidney; and procoagulative states like pregnancy, protein S and C deficiency, antithrombin III deficiency and contraceptive pills. The portal vein is patent so the diagnosis is not portal vein thrombosis, although the two conditions may present in almost the same manner. In this case liver failure looks imminent and prompt referral to a liver unit should be undertaken. Ecstasy overdose can cause acute liver failure but not after 3 weeks.

4.38 D* This patient has a radiculopathy at S1, possibly due to a prolapsed intervertebral disc. The hallmark of nerve root disease is pain that may start in the back and radiate down the buttock and leg. Myopathy usually presents as a bilateral symmetrical (proximal) weakness without sensory loss. Peripheral neuropathy typically presents as distal and asymmetrical weakness with fasciculation and sensory loss. Myelopathy/spinal cord disease presents with spastic paraparesis causing symmetrical distal muscle weakness. There may also be a sensory level below which there is a decrease in sensation. Similarly, there may be bowel and bladder symptoms. Subcortical lesions would cause a complete hemiparesis affecting the face, arm and leg.

4.39 C* Only 10–35% of patients with lung carcinoma have tumours that are surgically resectable. Contraindications include distant metastases involving the liver, brain and spine. Mediastinal spread includes: left recurrent laryngeal nerve involvement (which may result in hoarse voice), oesophagus (dysphagia), pericardium, phrenic nerve (causing high hemidiaphragm) and Horner's syndrome. Hypercalcaemia if not due to metastases is not a contraindication to surgery. Lung function tests are performed to assess the patient's ability to withstand thoracotomy pre- and postoperatively. Preoperatively the FEV_1 and FVC should be >50% of predicted, however, patients may survive the operation if the predicted postoperative FEV_1 is >0.8L.

4.40 C* This man presents with urethritis, migratory arthritis, skin rash and tenosynovitis. He has multiple sexual partners, which would make him at risk of contracting gonorrhoea. Gonococcal arthritis is more common in females than males. Failure to identify the organism in the joint fluid (up to 80%) does not exclude the diagnosis. Palindromic rheumatoid arthritis is a differential diagnosis for polyarticular arthritis but it is not usually migratory and is not associated with urethritis or skin rash.

4.41 B* The X-ray shows a drawing pin in the right lung as the cause of her condition, ruling out the other plausible options.

4.42 B* The chest X-ray shows a mass that extends into the neck. Teratoma and thymoma do not extend into the neck. This cannot be a thoracic aortic aneurysm as there is a normal aortic knuckle. Hodgkin's lymphoma would be unlikely as there is no hilar involvement.

4.43 A** The photograph of this young boy shows a scar with poor healing, which could be confused for keloid but the associated features are characteristic of Ehlers–Danlos syndrome (EDS). EDS is an inherited disorder of elastic tissue and is associated with increased joint mobility and skin fragility and hyper-extensibility. Pseudoxanthoma elasticum involves degeneration and calcification of the elastic fibres of the eyes, skin and arteries. It is associated with cutis laxa, where the skin appears wrinkled and sagging rather than breaking easily.

4.44 E* This patient presents with progressive shortness of breath and signs of right heart failure; chest X-ray shows a normal-sized heart with no evidence of pulmonary oedema. The two main differential diagnoses are restrictive cardiomyopathy and constrictive pericarditis. Restrictive cardiomyopathy is a primary myocardial disease characterised by rigid, non-compliant ventricular walls that resist diastolic filling. It may be caused by diffuse infiltration of the myocardium by amyloidosis (of which rheumatoid arthritis is a predisposing condition). Dilated cardiomyopathy would result in a large heart with dilatation of all chambers; there would be cardiomegaly on chest X-ray. With hypertrophic cardiomyopathy, patients would present younger and usually with systolic murmurs due to outflow tract obstruction.

4.45 E** This patient with Crohn's disease presents with abdominal pain rather than diarrhoea. A colonoscopy shows extensive large bowel involvement. He may have subacute small bowel obstruction due to small bowel involvement. The best test that would show this would be a small bowel enema or follow-through. A radiolabelled white cell scan may help in localising areas of inflammation that appear normal on colonoscopy.

4.46 D** Seizures are classified as partial, if they are confined to one cerebral hemisphere, or generalised, if they involve both hemispheres. Partial seizures can be further subdivided into simple, if consciousness is not impaired, or complex, if there is loss of consciousness. This patient has simple partial seizures associated with an aura. Absence seizures, myoclonic and tonic-clonic seizures are generalised seizures.

4.47 B** This patient has an obstructive lung function picture as the FEV_1:FVC ratio is 46%. All the other options would result in a restrictive pattern. The large TLC makes emphysema much more likely than chronic bronchitis.

4.48 A** Alkaptonuria or ochronosis is a rare defect in tyrosine catabolism due to deficiency of homogentisic acid oxidase. Patients present with degenerative arthritis, aortic stenosis, abnormal pigmentation and deposition of homogentisic acid in the sclera, ear and cochlea, leading to deafness. The arthritis may resemble ankylosing spondylitis but the X-ray findings do not show the annular ossification or sacroiliac joint fusion.

4.49 **C**** The X-ray appearances are that of bilateral bronchiectasis with dilated bronchi seen end on and longitudinally. There are many causes of bronchiectasis, including respiratory infections in childhood (particularly whooping cough, measles and tuberculosis), cystic fibrosis, hypogammaglobulinaemia states, bronchial obstruction conditions, fibrosis complicating lung infections, and allergic bronchopulmonary aspergillosis. COPD does not cause bronchiectasis.

4.50 **D*** This patient has a squamous cell carcinoma on top of his head. Recognised causes include sunlight and ultraviolet light exposure; radiation; chronic skin injury including burns and ulcers; chemical exposure, for example to arsenic; immunosuppression; and human papilloma virus. Pigmented naevi are associated with development of melanoma.

4.51 **D**** This patient has all the classical features of Klinefelter's syndrome of gynaecomastia, small testes and azoospermia. It is caused by an abnormal chromosome complement.

4.52 **C*** To diagnose hereditary non-polyposis colorectal cancer, three criteria have to be satisfied: there should be at least three relatives who have suffered from colorectal cancer; there should be involvement of two generations; and one of the individuals should be aged under 50. Familial adenomatous polyposis and Gardner's syndrome are associated with the development of multiple colonic adenomas.

4.53 **C*** MEN 1 syndrome is associated with hyperplasia or neoplastic transformation of the parathyroids, pancreatic islets and pituitary gland. This patient has a prolactinoma, developed hyperparathyroidism causing the peptic ulcer and a probable glucagonoma suggested by the necrolytic migratory erythema and diabetes.

4.54 **A**** A neoplasm maybe a possibility and certainly, if she had a change in bowel habit, anaemia and loss of weight, this would have to be excluded. However, she appears to have acute inflammation with some bleeding rectally so acute diverticulitis is the most likely diagnosis. Inflammatory bowel disease would be unusual in this age group. Pseudomembranous colitis may be considered if there was a history of antibiotic use.

4.55 **A**** This patient has a hyperosmolar non-ketotic (HONK) state (see **2.5**). The principles of treatment differ slightly from that of diabetic ketoacidosis. In diabetic ketoacidosis the main aim is to rehydrate, correct acidosis and prevent further ketosis. In HONK it is important to treat the underlying cause as well as rehydrate. Big shifts in the osmolality caused by large doses of insulin to bring down the blood glucose can lead to central pontine myelinolysis; far safer would be to have a small but constant infusion of intravenous insulin and then to use a 'sliding scale' insulin regimen when the blood glucose has come down gradually. Because of the high osmolality there is increased blood viscosity and so thromboembolism is a risk. Gastroparesis can also occur and nasogastric intubation therefore may be necessary to prevent aspiration. As such patients are not insulin dependent, they will remain diabetic but may not need tablets or insulin once recovered.

4.56 C* This patient has nephrocalcinosis, as suggested by the plain X-ray and the history of repeated stones. In this autosomal recessive condition the flow of urine is slowed from the tubules into the renal pelvis, leading to super-saturation of the urine and stone formation. RTA I is characterised by a defect in urinary acidification and renal ammoniagenesis, which results in a net accumulation of acids within body fluids. Unlike RTA II, where there is a failure to reabsorb bicarbonate ions in the proximal tubule, RTA I results in an inability to excrete H^+ ions in the distal tubule and so urinary pH is never <5.3. Other features of RTA I include association with renal parenchymal disease, such as medullary sponge kidney, normal anion gap and profound hypokalaemia due to increased exchange between Na^+ and K^+ ions at the distal tubule. Features of RTA II include variable urine pH, serum bicarbonate between 14–20, Fanconi's syndrome (hypophosphataemia, hyperuricaemia, glycosuria and volume depletion) and osteomalacia. RTA IV is associated with hyporeninaemic hypoaldosteronism, hyperkalaemia and diabetic nephropathy. Conn's syndrome is a cause of hypokalaemia associated with primary hyper-aldosteronism. Bartter's syndrome is a salt-losing state due to defective chloride reabsorption at the loop of Henle and is associated with hypokalaemia and hyperreninaemia.

4.57 B** The blood film shows a long nematode worm between blood cells. They may present with swellings on the limbs known as Calabar swellings.

4.58 C* This patient presents with symptoms of jaundice, conjunctivitis, anaemia and meningism following the onset of a flu-like illness after a camping trip. During that time she may have come into contact with contaminated water and contracted leptospirosis. If allowed to progress it may lead to hepatic failure, meningitis and renal failure. There may occasionally be a rash but this is non-specific. Rocky Mountain spotted fever and Lyme disease are both associated with a characteristic rash and do not cause liver dysfunction. Histoplasmosis may mimic tuberculosis but she has no chest signs and a clear chest X-ray. Hepatitis A does not usually cause conjunctivitis or meningitis.

4.59 A** The poor prognostic factors for Hodgkin's lymphoma include: male sex, lymphocyte-depleted disease, bulky mediastinal disease, older age, and development of B symptoms. B symptoms include unexplained fever, drench-ing night sweats and weight loss of >10% over 6 months. Subdiaphragmatic disease is associated with wider disseminated disease; in this case, the patient has disease on both sides of the diaphragm, giving her stage III disease according to the Ann Arbor staging system.

4.60 A* Alport's syndrome is an X-linked dominant disease where sensorineural deafness presents by age 7 and microscopic haematuria is usually present by age 10. Proteinuria and renal failure tend to develop well into adulthood. Ocular abnormalities can also occur and include myopia, retinintis pigmentosa, anterior lenticonus and cataracts. Urogenital investigations reveal no evidence of structural abnormalities. Juvenile nephronophthisis is an inherited tubulointerstitial nephropathy that eventually leads to renal failure and patients present with polyuria, polydipsia and weight loss, progressive loss of vision (secondary to retinal degeneration) and small, cystic, hyperechoic kidneys on ultrasound. Fabry's disease is an X-linked recessive deficiency of α-galactosidase A which leads to progressive haematuria, proteinuria, renal failure, skin lesions and peripheral neuropathy. Thin basement membrane disease is an autosomal dominant condition characterised by persistent microscopic haematuria but normal renal function. Autosomal dominant polycystic kidney disease tends to present with loin pain, haematuria, renal dysfunction, hypertension, nephrolithiasis and recurrent urinary tract infections; there may also be extrarenal complications, including liver cysts and fibrosis, intracranial and aortic aneurysms, colonic diverticula and pancreatic cysts.

Paper 5

Questions

5.1 A 67-year-old male patient on the ward developed severe central chest pain that did not respond to glyceryl trinitrate. He had been admitted 2 days ago with progressive shortness of breath on exertion but no chest pain. The pain radiated up to the neck and he felt nauseous. He had a previous medical history of hypertension and chronic renal failure. His only medication was furosemide (frusemide) and enalapril. He smoked 20 cigarettes per day and drank 2 units of alcohol per week. There was a family history of myocardial infarction.

On examination he was in pain, looked unwell and was sweating. His temperature was 36.6°C, pulse 100 regular and blood pressure 150/88. His JVP was not elevated, his heart sounds were normal with no murmurs but he did have bilateral crackles in his chest. Abdominal examination was normal.

Bloods				
	Hb	12.0	WCC	9.3
	Platelets	400	Na	143
	K	4.1	Urea	15.4
	Creatinine	220	Glucose	4.2
	Magnesium	0.86		

Chest X-ray Some upper lobe blood diversion

No pulmonary oedema

ECG T wave inversion V_{4-6} present on admission

The patient was suspected of having an acute coronary syndrome/non Q-wave MI.

The most important diagnostic test to enable urgent further treatment would be:

A development of RBBB on further ECG
B serum CK-MB
C serum LDH
D serum troponin T and I
E urgent echocardiogram

5.2 A 73-year-old man was referred with collapse.

His ECG (see following page) shows:

    A 1st degree AV block
    B complete heart block
    C Mobitz type I 2nd degree AV block
    D Mobitz type II 2nd degree AV block
    E sinus bradycardia

5.3   A 19-year-old girl was admitted with difficulty in swallowing; 36 hours previously she had taken an overdose of metoclopramide. Over the last 3 hours she had developed progressively worse dysphagia and drooling. She also complained of blurred vision.

    On examination she was distressed but alert. There was drooping of the left side of her mouth. Her left eye was deviated to the left. The rest of her cranial nerve examination was normal. The treatment of choice for this patient is:

    A adrenaline (epinephrine)
    B chlorphenamine (chlorpheniramine)
    C hydrocortisone
    D prochlorperazine
    E procyclidine

5.4   A 37-year-old woman was admitted with headache, fever, neck stiffness and malaise. She had also noticed a non-pruritic rash on her left leg, which had got progressively bigger. Two weeks ago she had returned with her family from a camping holiday in the USA. No one else in her family was ill. She had no previous medical problems and was not on any medication.

    On examination she had a temperature of 38.3°C and bilateral, tender, cervical lymphadenopathy. Her pulse was 92 regular and blood pressure 135/78. There was some tenderness in her lower limb joints but no swelling, erythema or effusions and she had normal range of movements. Cranial nerve examination was normal (Figure 5.4). See plate section.

The skin rash is most likely:

    A erythema chronicum migrans
    B erythema gyratum repens
    C erythema marginatum
    D erythema nodosum
    E granuloma annulare

5.5   A 45-year-old man presented with worsening chest pain that came on with exertion. He was a smoker and drank 5 units of alcohol per day. He had no other medical problems and was not on any medication.

    He was rather obese on examination. His pulse was 80 regular and his blood pressure was 130/80.

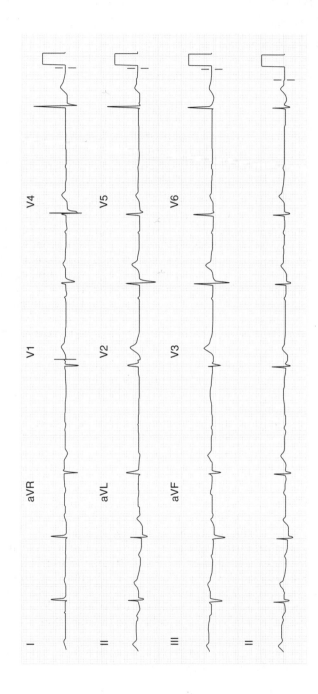

Bloods	Glucose	12.0	TSH	2.5
	Free T$_4$	20.5	Cholesterol	3.5
	Triglycerides	35	LDL cholesterol	2.7
	HDL cholesterol	0.8		

Aside from lifestyle changes, the drug treatment of choice would be:

A bezafibrate
B colestyramine
C nicotinic acid
D simvastatin
E thyroxine

5.6 A large randomised control trial comparing aspirin to warfarin in preventing recurrence of ischaemic stroke was published. All 2000 patients had a previous history of ischaemic stroke, of whom 1000 patients were male. The age ranges for the two groups were similar. Randomisation was determined by the toss of a coin. All patients received the same care apart from the drug being investigated. There were equal numbers of withdrawals from both groups. Both groups' data was analysed in exactly the same way and on an intention to treat basis. A significant reduction in recurrence of stroke in the warfarin group (absolute risk reduction 10%; 95% confidence interval 120 to 443) was found.

The **ONE** type of bias which flaws this study is:

A Detection bias
B Exclusion bias
C Performance bias
D Recall bias
E Selection bias

5.7 A 55-year-old women was referred with recurrent upper abdominal pain. The pain was worse after eating and came and went rapidly. Appetite was normal and there was no weight loss. There was no previous medical history or significant family history. She drank 2 units of alcohol at the weekend and smoked 20 cigarettes per day.
   On examination there was no jaundice or anaemia and she did not appear dehydrated. Her temperature was 37 2°C, pulse 95 regular and blood pressure 130/85. There was diffuse upper abdominal tenderness with no organomegaly and normal rectal examination.

Bloods	Hb	13.9	WCC	12.5
	Platelets	300	INR	1.1
	Na	141	K	4.9
	Urea	4.5	Creatinine	75

	Bilirubin	20		Protein	65
	Albumin	38		ALT	120
	ALP	145		GGT	90
	Amylase	100			

Chest X-ray Normal

Abdominal X-ray Normal

The most helpful and appropriate investigation for establishing the diagnosis would be:

    A abdominal ultrasound
    B antiendomysial antibodies
    C barium meal
    D CT abdomen
    E upper GI endoscopy

5.8   A 14-year-old Afro-Caribbean boy presented with severe abdominal pain and shortness of breath for 1 day. He was known to suffer from sickle cell anaemia and had had similar attacks before but could not remember how they were treated. He was on no medication and had no other medical problems.

    On examination he was in pain and jaundiced. His temperature was 37.5°C, pulse 100 regular and blood pressure 98/60. His respiratory rate was 22 breaths/min and his chest was clear. He had tender hepatomegaly with no lymphadenopathy or ascites. There was no pain in his limbs. Neurological examination was normal.

Bloods	Hb	3.5		MCV	60.2
	WCC	4.0		Platelets	320
	Reticulocytes	18%		Na	135
	K	4.0		Urea	3.3
	Creatinine	70		Protein	65
	Albumin	35		Bilirubin	80
	ALT	25		ALP	345

Chest X-ray Normal

The type of crisis this patient is having is:

    A acute chest syndrome
    B aplastic
    C haemolytic
    D infarctive
    E sequestration

5.9 A 49-year-old man was referred with shortness of breath on exertion associated with a non-productive cough. He had normal exercise tolerance and no cardiac history. He had a normal appetite and no loss of weight. He had smoked 15 cigarettes a day for over 20 years. He had no other medical problems, was on no medication and had not travelled abroad recently.

On examination he was apyrexial, pulse 79 regular and blood pressure 138/88. His respiratory rate was 18 breaths/min and his chest sounded clear.

Chest X-ray   Right hilar lymphadenopathy

Lymph node biopsy   (Figure 5.9). See plate section.

The most likely diagnosis is:

   A lymphoma
   B lung carcinoma
   C reactive lymphadenopathy
   D tuberculosis
   E sarcoidosis

5.10 A 25-year-old woman had a routine screening blood test prior to starting a new job as a health care worker. She was fit and well.

HBsAg	Positive
HBeAg	Negative
Total anti-HBc	Positive
IgM anti-HBc	Negative
Anti-HBe	Positive
HBV DNA	Negative

The blood results are most compatible with:

   A acute hepatitis B infection
   B chronic hepatitis B carrier
   C chronic hepatitis B carrier who is actively replicating virus
   D immune to hepatitis B
   E vaccinated against hepatitis B

5.11 A 60-year-old woman presented with progressive fatigue and weakness. She found writing a real struggle and had had to reduce her activities. However, there was no paresthesiae and her symptoms improved with rest. She also complained of some double vision, dysphagia and shortness of breath on exertion. She had had no recent illnesses.

On examination she had bilateral ptosis and strabismus. Her face lacked expression and her voice was weak and nasal. The rest of her cranial nerve examination was normal. Her pulse was 72 regular and blood pressure was 120/80. Respiratory examination was normal. There was no limb muscle wasting or weakness. Tone, power, reflexes and sensation in upper and lower limbs were normal.

The test that would give the definitive diagnosis is:

A anti-Jo1 antibodies
B edrophonium (tensilon) test
C muscle biopsy
D nerve conduction studies
E temporal artery biopsy

5.12 A 55-year-old woman was referred with blurred vision. Fundoscopy was performed and is shown below (Figure 5.12). See plate section.

The fundoscopic appearance is most likely due to:

A choroidoretintits
B hypertensive retinopathy
C optic atrophy
D retinal artery occlusion
E retinitis pigmentosa

5.13 A 20-year-old known asthmatic man was brought in short of breath. Three days ago he developed a sore throat and cough productive of white sputum. Since then he had become increasingly short of breath and was using his inhalers much more frequently. His asthma had been well controlled and he had never been admitted to hospital because of his asthma. He did not have a nebuliser at home. The ambulance crew had put him on high flow oxygen and given him three nebules of salbutamol. He had been in treated in casualty for over an hour with another three nebules of salbutamol 5 mg (with oxygen) and 200 mg of hydrocortisone but with no improvement in his clinical state.

On examination he was panting and sitting forward. He was unable to complete a sentence or perform a peak flow. His temperature was 37.8°C, pulse 120 regular and blood pressure 95/60. There was intercostal recession, his respiratory rate was 36 breaths per minute and soft bilateral wheeze was heard.

Bloods	Hb	14.6	WCC	10.5
	Platelets	368	Neutrophils	5.5
	Na	140	K	3.9
	Urea	3.9	Creatinine	65

Blood gases on 60% O_2	pH	7.29	PCO_2	6.0
	PO_2	8.2	Bicarbonate	25
	Base excess	−5.6		

Chest X-ray (portable)	Normal			

The **LEAST** appropriate step in the immediate management of this patient would be to:

- A ask the anaesthetist to consider mechanical ventilation
- B increase the frequency of salbutamol nebulisers to every 10 minutes
- C give intravenous benzylpenicillin and clarithromycin
- D give intravenous magnesium sulphate
- E give intravenous salbutamol infusion

5.14 A 67-year-old woman was admitted with melaena having passed 500 mL of black stools. She had no abdominal pain, was not on non-steroidal anti-inflammatory drugs or anticoagulants and did not drink alcohol. Her only previous medical problems were intermittent dysphagia and arthritis affecting her hands. Last year Raynaud's phenomenon was diagnosed, following which she gave up smoking. Her only medication was ranitidine.

On examination she looked pale. She has telangiectasia on her face, lips and neck. Her pulse was 98 regular and blood pressure 150/90 with no postural drop on standing. Respiratory examination was normal. Abdomen was soft and tender. Rectal examination confirmed melaena. The skin of her hands was thickened and rough and her fingers were thin and spindly. The wrist and finger joints were tender but not obviously inflamed and she had normal range of movements.

Bloods					
Hb	9.8		MCV	73.6
WCC	7.9		Platelets	450
Na	145		K	4.2
Urea	8.7		Creatinine	145
Protein	70		Albumin	35
Bilirubin	12		ALT	16
ALP	56		ESR	35
CRP	28			

Rheumatoid factor	Negative
Antinuclear antibody	1 in 80
Anti-DS DNA	Negative
Anticentromere antibody	1 in 80
Anti-SCL 70 antibody	Negative
Anti-Ro antibody	Negative
Anti-La antibody	Negative
Anti-Jo1 antibody	Negative
Upper GI endoscopy	Normal oesophagus Telangiectasia in stomach

The most likely diagnosis is:

A amyloidosis
B CREST syndrome (calcinosis cutis, Raynaud's phenomenon, oesophageal dysfunction, sclerodactyly, telangiectasia)
C hereditary haemorrhagic telangiectasia
D Sjögren's syndrome
E systemic sclerosis

5.15 A 45-year-old man was referred for endoscopy because of indigestion (Figure 5.15). See plate section.

The endoscopic findings are consistent with:

A Barrett's oesophagus
B benign oesophageal stricture
C oesophageal candidasis
D oesophageal varices
E Schatzki ring

5.16 A 62-year-old man presented with collapse. His GCS score at the time of presentation was 14/15 (Figure 5.16). See plate section.

The CT scan shows:

A hydrocephalus
B left extradural haematoma
C left intracerebral haemorrhage
D left subdural haematoma
E subarachnoid haemorrhage

5.17 A 35-year-old HIV-positive man presented with headaches. He had no neck stiffness or personality change.
     On examination he had a temperature of 38.1°C and cervical lymphadenopathy. There was no rash. His pulse was 88 regular and blood pressure 120/78. Chest examination was normal. Fundoscopy and cranial nerve examination were normal.

Chest X-ray   Normal (Figure 5.17). See plate section

This patient should be started on:

A aciclovir
B cefotaxime
C co-trimoxazole
D dexamethasone
E pyrimethamine and sulfadiazine

5.18 A 15-year-old boy was referred because he found that he became short of breath when he tried to play football with his friends. He had to stop after only a few minutes and this was getting progressively worse. He had no previous medical problems and was not on any medication.

On examination he looked well and was not cyanosed. His pulse was 75 regular and blood pressure 120/72. His JVP was just visible and he had a fixed split second heart sound. There was a systolic murmur, loudest at the left upper sternal edge. The apex was not displaced. Respiratory examination was normal.

ECG   RBBB

           Right axis deviation

           No ischaemic changes

The most likely diagnosis is:

A hypertrophic obstructive cardiomyopathy (HOCM)
B ostium primum atrial septal defect
C ostium secundum atrial septal defect
D patent ductus arteriosus
E ventricular septal defect

5.19 A 64-year-old man presented with acute diplopia, dysphagia and dysarthria. He suffered from diabetes and hypertension. He had never had these symptoms before.

On examination he had a right Horner's syndrome. There was decreased temperature and pinprick sensation on the right side of the face. There was right-sided palatal paralysis with absent gag reflex. He had right-sided ataxia and nystagmus. There was no dysphasia but some dysarthria. There was normal tone, power and reflexes in the upper and lower limbs but decreased pinprick sensation on the left upper and lower limbs.

The blood vessel most likely to be occluded is:

A basilar artery
B middle cerebral artery
C posterior cerebral artery
D posterior inferior cerebellar artery
E superior cerebellar artery

5.20 A 45-year-old man was referred because of a 3-day history of severe pain in his right middle finger (Figure 5.20). See plate section.

The most likely diagnosis is

    A Heberden's node
    B rheumatoid nodule
    C septic arthritis
    D tophaceous gout
    E scleroderma

5.21 A 75-year-old Caucasian woman suffered a fall at home. Her daughter was concerned whether she had osteoporosis. A DEXA scan was performed and she has returned wanting to know the result.

DEXA scan of total hip T score   −0.8

                                   Z score   −0.5

The interpretation of the DEXA scan result is:

    A normal bone mass
    B osteopenia appropriate for her age
    C osteopenia inappropriate for her age
    D osteoporosis appropriate for her age
    E osteoporosis inappropriate for her age

5.22 A 35-year-old woman who was 27 weeks pregnant was admitted with severe headache and blurred vision. She reported no neck stiffness or photophobia. She had no previous medical problems and this was her first pregnancy and up until now she had had no complications. She was on no medication.

    On examination she had a temperature of 38.1°C, pulse 100 regular and blood pressure 100/68. Chest and heart sounds were normal. Abdomen was distended consistent with pregnancy. There was no focal neurological defect and plantar responses were flexor. She had widespread purpuric lesions on her back and lower limbs. There was no peripheral oedema.

Bloods	Hb	8.0	MCV	106.2
	WCC	23.2	Neutrophils	19.1
	Platelets	35	Reticulocytes	13%
	INR	1.0	Na	137
	K	4.4	Urea	35.3
	Creatinine	300	Protein	68
	Albumin	37	Bilirubin	35
	ALT	20	ALP	96
	GGT	50		
Blood film	Red cell fragments			
Chest X-ray	Normal			

The most likely diagnosis is:

A disseminated intravascular coagulopathy
B fatty liver of pregnancy
C HELLP syndrome (haemolytic anaemia, elevated liver enzymes and low platelets)
D thrombotic thrombocytopenic purpura
E toxic shock syndrome

5.23 It had been proposed that helical CT chest could be used to screen for lung carcinoma. A trial using 500 patients was carried out 140 cases of carcinoma developed. The CT detected 60 cases and 25 false-positives.

The specificity of CT as a screening test is:

A 60/85
B 60/140
C 335/360
D 335/415
E 395/500

5.24 A 64-year-old woman with osteoarthritis presented with a several month history of lethargy and itching, which kept her awake at night. She had decreased appetite but had been putting on weight, which she attributed to her abdomen becoming larger.

On examination there were scratch marks over her forearms and legs. She had moderate ascites and 3 cm hepatomegaly.

Bloods				
	Hb	12.4	WCC	5.7
	Platelets	100	Bilirubin	38
	Albumin	32	Protein	69
	ALT	40	ALP	170
	GGT	120		

The **SINGLE** most effective drug for treatment of her pruritus would be:

A azathioprine
B chlorphenamine (chlorpheniramine)
C colestyramine
D penicillamine
E prednisolone

5.25 A 16-year-old boy presented with 3-day history of bleeding gums and generalised purpura. On examination he had a temperature of 39.1°C. He had bilateral cervical lymphadenopathy and palpable splenomegaly.

Bloods   Hb   13.1   WCC   2.9

              Platelets   30

Blood film   Atypical lymphocytes

The most likely diagnosis is:

   A acute lymphoblastic leukaemia
   B acute myeloid leukaemia
   C aplastic anaemia
   D Henoch–Schönlein purpura
   E infectious mononucleosis

5.26 A 25-year-old HIV-positive man was admitted with bloody diarrhoea that had been going on for 3 weeks. He had a decreased appetite and some weight loss. He was not on any medication. He contracted HIV from an infected needle but was hepatitis B and C negative. He did not drink alcohol but did smoke.

     On examination he looked thin. His temperature was 37.3°C, pulse 88 regular and blood pressure 130/89. His chest was clear. His abdomen was generally tender with no organomegaly. Rectal examination revealed no masses.

Chest X-ray   Normal

Colonoscopy was performed and biopsies were taken (Figure 5.26). See plate section.

The most likely diagnosis is:

   A cytomegalovirus colitis
   B giardiasis
   C Kaposi's sarcoma
   D *Mycobacterium avium intracellulare* complex
   E *Mycobacterium* TB

5.27 A 36-year-old female was referred to the neurologist from Accident & Emergency with a provisional diagnosis of deliberate self-harm because she kept burning herself with cigarettes. She denied any suicidal ideation but felt depressed that she had no pain sensation in her hands, which were ugly and deformed. She had no previous medical history and no family history of note. She was a heavy smoker.

     On examination she had right Horner's syndrome and mild kyphosis of her spine. There was no cyanosis or lymphadenopathy. There was wasting of the small muscles of her hands and tone, power and reflexes in her upper limbs was decreased. There was loss of pinprick sensation but intact light touch and vibration sense. In her legs there was increased tone, some muscle weakness, increased reflexes and extensor plantars but she was able to walk. Cranial nerve examination was normal. Examination of the cardiovascular and respiratory systems revealed no abnormality. The most likely diagnosis is:

A cervical myelopathy
B Charcot–Marie–Tooth disease (HSMN)
C motor neurone disease
D Pancoast's tumour
E syringomyelia

5.28 A 68-year-old woman who was known to have COPD was admitted with shortness of breath. She was on home nebulisers of salbutamol and ipratropium bromide but not home oxygen. Her last admission with the same problem was 6 months ago and she had never required ventilation. Today she had used her nebuliser four times without relief. The ambulance crew had given her another two nebules plus oxygen.

On examination in Accident & Emergency she was on 40% oxygen. She was drowsy. Her temperature was 36.9°C, pulse 120 regular and blood pressure 130/80. Respiratory rate was 26 breaths per minute but she was unable to talk in full sentences. She had bilateral wheeze in her chest.

Arterial blood gases on 40% O_2	pH	7.25	PCO_2	10.5
	PO_2	9.5	Bicarbonate	34
	Base excess	6.2	O_2 saturation	90%

Chest X-ray No pneumothorax or consolidation. Hyperinflated lungs

The next most appropriate immediate management step would be to:

A increase the oxygen to 60% with a rebreathing bag and repeat arterial blood gases in 30 minutes
B reduce the oxygen to 28% and repeat arterial blood gases in 30 minutes
C start a doxapram infusion
D start non-invasive partial pressure ventilation
E start on oral prednisolone and oral antibiotics

5.29 A 45-year-old man was referred with bilateral paresthesiae up to mid-shin that had been present for 3 months. He also complained of pain in his hips and knees and had a purpuric rash on his legs. He used to be an intravenous drug abuser and 6 months ago had become jaundiced, which had resolved spontaneously.

On examination he was not in pain. His temperature was 36.5°C, pulse 78 regular and blood pressure 147/76. Respiratory examination was normal. He had mild abdominal tenderness but no organomegaly. He had decreased sensation to light touch and pinprick up to the level of mid-shin. There was normal lower limb tone and power but absent ankle and plantar reflexes.

Bloods	Hb	11.9	MCV	92.4
	WCC	7.6	Platelets	459
	Na	138	K	4.8

Urea	10.8	Creatinine	130
Protein	74	Albumin	38
Bilirubin	15	ALT	55
ALP	100	ESR	65
CRP	58	C3	70
C4	30		

Rheumatoid factor   Negative

Antinuclear antibody   Negative

ANCA   Negative

Hepatitis A, C serology Negative

Hepatitis B serology   HBsAg positive
                                  HBeAg positive

Chest X-ray   Normal

The most likely diagnosis is:

     A   microscopic polyangitis
     B   mixed cryoglobulinaemia
     C   polyarteritis nodosa
     D   systemic lupus erythematosus
     E   Wegener's granulomatosis

5.30 This 45-year-old man was referred because of nodules that had developed on his right forearm 2 weeks after cleaning out his aquarium. On examination he was apyrexial (Figure 5.30). See plate section.

The most likely diagnosis is:

     A   anthrax
     B   Herpes simplex
     C   molluscum contagiosum
     D   *Mycobacterium marinum*
     E   orf

5.31 A 59-year-old man presented with a 5-month history of frontal headaches (Figure 5.31). See plate section.

The most likely diagnosis is:

     A   acromegaly
     B   hyperparathyroidism
     C   hypophysis tumour
     D   multiple myeloma
     E   Paget's disease of bone

5.32 A 50-year-old man was referred by his general practitioner for a barium swallow and meal. He had found him to be anaemic on a routine blood count (Figure 5.32). See plate section.

The most likely diagnosis is:

    A achalasia
    B benign stricture
    C carcinoma of the oesophagus
    D oesophageal candidiasis
    E oesophageal varices

5.33 A 14-year-old boy was referred with worsening syncopal episodes. He had a heart murmur at birth and an operation soon afterwards. He became very short of breath with exercise.

    On examination there was finger clubbing and central cyanosis. There was a thoracotomy scar. His pulse was 88 regular and blood pressure 100/76. The left radial pulse was weaker than the right radial pulse. There was a left parasternal heave and a systolic thrill at the left upper sternal edge accompanied by a loud ejection systolic murmur. His chest was clear.

Which **ONE** of the following statements is likely to be true of this patient's condition?

    A β-Blockers are the drug treatment of choice
    B He has pulmonary hypertension due to development of Eisenmenger's syndrome
    C Squatting would make his symptoms worse
    D Syncope is due to left-to-right intracardiac shunting of blood
    E Syncope is likely to be due to dislodged vegetations from infective endocarditis

5.34 A 56-year-old woman had an emergency operation for a ruptured aortic aneurysm; 4 hours postoperatively she became tachycardic and hypotensive. While talking to the doctor who had been asked to see her she lost consciousness. He could not feel a pulse or hear any breath sounds. The cardiac monitor showed the following trace:

The next step in the immediate management of this patient would be:

  A adrenaline (epinephrine) I mg intravenously
  B defibrillate 200 J
  C lidocaine (lignocaine) 100 mg intravenously
  D precordial thump
  E start cardiopulmonary chest compressions

5.35 A 63-year-old man had just returned from a holiday in India. His previous medical history included non-insulin dependent diabetes mellitus, hypertension and atrial fibrillation, for which he was on a number of medications (Figure 5.35). See plate section.

The most likely cause of his skin rash is:

  A atenolol
  B digoxin
  C gliclazide
  D hydrochlorothiazide
  E metformin

5.36 A 65-year-old woman presented with a 2-month history of a painless swelling in her neck. It was getting bigger but not causing problems with swallowing or breathing. She had a normal appetite and no weight loss. She had no previous medical history and was not on any medication.

On examination there was a 3 cm firm, non-tender single nodule in her thyroid gland. There was no associated lymphadenopathy or goitre. She was clinically euthyroid.

Bloods   TSH   1.6   Free T$_4$ 20

The next most appropriate investigation in this patient would be:

  A CT thoracic inlet
  B fine needle aspiration of the nodule
  C flow–volume loop
  D radioisotope scan
  E ultrasound of the thyroid

5.37 You have been asked to sit on the research and development committee to consider a research application for a screening test for Creutzfeldt–Jakob disease. It is claimed that CJD patients who present with myoclonic jerks have abnormally high levels of enzyme x in their blood. The prevalence is estimated to be 1 in 20,000 and the test is estimated to have a specificity of 90% and a sensitivity of 92%.

The major flaw with this screening test is that:

A it would be too harmful to the patient
B the disease is too rare
C the test is too difficult to measure
D the test will be too expensive
E the test will not alter management

5.38 A 45-year-old man presented with a 2-day history of worsening severe central abdominal pain. He had vomited four times but had no haematemesis. The pain was like a knife and radiated to the back; movement made his symptoms worse. He had not opened his bowels today. He also suffered from ulcerative colitis. His inflammatory bowel disease was difficult to control and he was on azathioprine and mesalazine and a course of prednisolone. He drank 4 units of alcohol a day and smoked 10 cigarettes a day.

On examination he was in severe pain. He had a temperature of 38.2°C and he looked pale. His pulse was 110 regular and blood pressure 98/59. His abdomen was distended and there was rebound tenderness and generalised guarding. Bowel sounds were absent.

Bloods	Hb	11.5	WCC	25.4
	Neutrophils	22.8	Platelets	345
	Na	135	K	4.0
	Urea	7.8	Creatinine	150
	Bilirubin	25	ALT	35
	ALP	95	GGT	130
	Albumin	33	Phosphate	0.7

Chest X-ray Free air under the right hemidiaphragm

Abdominal X-ray No obstruction

Which **ONE** of the following statements concerning this patient's condition is true?

A A fall in the haematocrit greater than 10% after 48 hours carries a worse prognosis
B A serum amylase >2000 has a poor prognosis
C ERCP should be performed as soon as possible
D Hypocalcaemia is a cause of this patient's symptoms
E Urgent laparotomy should be performed if he fails to improve within the first 72 hours

5.39 A 69-year-old woman was admitted with dysarthria and dysphagia of sudden onset. She was known to suffer from atrial fibrillation and had had several minor strokes affecting both sides. There was a family history of stroke and she smoked 20 cigarettes per day.

On examination she had no facial abnormalities. She was able to name objects and follow commands. Her speech was slow and indistinct. She was unable to protrude her tongue, which was small and tight. Saliva dribbled persistently from her mouth. The corneal reflex was intact. The jaw jerk appeared brisk. The gag reflex was intact. The patient is most likely to have:

A bulbar palsy
B cerebellopontine angle lesion
C jugular foramen syndrome
D medial medullary syndrome
E pseudobulbar palsy

5.40 A 55-year-old man was referred for lung function tests because of shortness of breath and chronic cough. His flow–volume loop is most consistent with:

A asthma
B emphysema
C fibrosing alveolitis
D normality
E retrosternal goitre

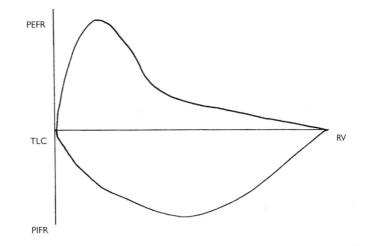

5.41 A 28-year-old man presented with a 3-week history of pain and stiffness in his right ankle; no other joints were affected. A month ago he had had conjunctivitis involving the right eye, which had resolved spontaneously. He also had a painless ulcer on his penis and some discomfort when he passed urine. He was heterosexual and had multiple sexual partners.

On examination his temperature was 37.2°C, pulse 88 regular and blood pressure 130/74. Respiratory and abdominal systems were normal. The right ankle was swollen and tender. There was also some thickening and tenderness of the Achilles' tendon. His other leg and hands were normal and there was no skin rash.

Bloods

Hb	12.0	WCC	11.8
Neutrophils	8.8	Platelets	480
Na	137	K	4.2
Urea	5.7	Creatinine	89
Protein	70	Albumin	40
Bilirubin	10	ALT	25
ALP	70	ESR	34
CRP	40		

Synovial fluid Slightly turbid appearance

WCC	35000	Neutrophils	60%

No growth

Protein 35

Urine culture No growth

The most likely diagnosis is

- A ankylosing spondylitis
- B Behçet's syndrome
- C gonococcal arthritis
- D Reiter's syndrome
- E rheumatoid arthritis

5.42 This 50-year-old woman was referred with a 3-month history of burning in both ears that came and went, and was associated with deafness and vertigo. She also had a deformity of her nose and in the past suffered from episcleritis and arthritis of the shoulder and hip (Figure 5.42). See plate section.

The most likely diagnosis is:

- A Reiter's syndrome
- B relapsing polychondritis
- C syphilis
- D systemic lupus erythematosus
- E Wegener's granulomatosis

5.43 A 45-year-old woman presented with collapse. Her GCS score at the time of presentation was 14/15 (Figure 5.43). See plate section.

The CT scan shows:

    A left cerebral infarct
    B left extradural haematoma
    C left intracerebral haemorrhage
    D left subdural haematoma
    E subarachnoid haemorrhage

5.44 A 16-year-old boy was admitted with a 3-day history of malaise, abdominal pain and microscopic haematuria. He was on no medication. Further to this he had now developed a non-pruritic rash affecting his lower limbs (Figure 5.44). See plate section.

His temperature was 37.4°C, pulse 88 regular and blood pressure 110/88. He had generalised abdominal tenderness and urine dipstick was positive for red cells and protein.

Which **ONE** of the following statements concerning this patient's condition is **TRUE**?

    A He is at risk of developing haemolytic uraemic syndrome
    B He is likely to have a low platelet count
    C He should be started on high dose intravenous antibiotics immediately
    D Intravenous hydrocortisone should be given
    E Skin biopsy would provide the definitive diagnosis

5.45 A 40-year-old woman was admitted with weakness, paresthesiae, muscle cramps, headaches and palpitations. Her symptoms had been getting worse over the past month. She had no previous medical history. She did not smoke or drink alcohol.

On examination her pulse was 90 regular and blood pressure 190/105. Her JVP was not elevated and heart sounds and chest examination were normal. Abdominal examination was normal.

Bloods	Na	137	K	2.9
	Urea	5.5	Creatinine	98
	Glucose	5.9	Magnesium	0.69
	Bicarbonate	37		

The most appropriate treatment pending investigation for her hypertension is:

    A methyldopa
    B nifedipine
    C phenoxybenzamine
    D propanolol
    E spironolactone

5.46 A 29-year-old man presented with a 4-week history of abdominal pain and bloody diarrhoea. He opened his bowels up to five times per day and his stools were liquid, containing fresh blood. He had not eaten anything unusual nor been abroad recently. He had a decreased appetite and had lost over 3 kg in weight. He had no previous medical history and there was no relevant family history.

On examination he looked ill and had a temperature of 38.0°C. His pulse was 110 regular and blood pressure 95/60. Chest examination was normal. His abdomen was very tender and distended. Rectal examination revealed bloody stool.

Bloods	Hb	10.4	WCC	13.5
	Platelets	450	INR	1.0
	Na	138	K	3.9
	Urea	7.5	Creatinine	100
	Albumin	28	Bilirubin	12
	Protein	60	ALT	20
	ALP	65	Amylase	30
	Calcium	2.20	Phosphate	0.8
	ESR	65	CRP	250

The next most appropriate investigation of this patient would be:

A abdominal ultrasound
B abdominal X-ray
C barium enema
D CT abdomen
E flexible sigmoidoscopy

5.47 A 33-year-old man was brought to Accident & Emergency with generalised fits. They had started 20 minutes ago and had continued despite the patient being given 2×10 mg of diazepam intravenously. He had associated tongue biting and jerking of all limbs. He was not conscious and did not respond to commands. He had no previous medical history of epilepsy.

On examination he had a temperature of 38.5°C, pulse 110 regular and blood pressure 150/90 when he briefly stopped fitting. His chest sounded clear. Pupils responded to light and his plantar responses were bilaterally extensor.

Bloods	Hb	14.4	WCC	12.3
	Platelets	160	Na	138
	K	4.0	Urea	4.9
	Creatinine	89	Glucose	5.6
	Calcium	2.1	Magnesium	0.8
	Protein	70	Albumin	40

Which **ONE** of the following statements is correct?

A Bilateral extensor plantars are consistent with a permanent intracranial event
B He should be restrained as he is at risk of hurting himself and other patients
C Intravenous sodium valproate should be considered next in his immediate management
D Lorazepam could be used just as effectively as diazepam
E Pyrexia, urine dipstick and microscopy showing blood but not haemoglobin are suggestive of an underlying urinary tract infection

5.48 A 69-year-old lady presented to her general practitioner with low back pain that had been getting progressively worse over the past 3 months.

Which **ONE** of the following symptoms would suggest her condition was due to an infiltrative, non-inflammatory cause?

A Activity makes her back pain worse
B Her back pain is only felt down one side
C Her symptoms are unaffected by change in position and not improved by supine position with hips flexed
D There is associated morning stiffness lasting more than I hour
E There is nocturnal pain

5.49 A 61-year-old woman presented with bloody diarrhoea that had been going on for 4 weeks. She had decreased appetite and had lost 3 kg in weight. She opened her bowels five times per day and twice at night and the stools were liquid with blood. She was not on any medication (Figure 5.49). See plate section.

The barium enema shows:

A Crohn's disease
B diverticulitis
C ischaemic colitis
D normal colon
E ulcerative colitis

5.50 A 32-year-old woman presented with a facial rash that had worsened over 6 weeks and was limited to the chin, cheeks and nose (Figure 5.50). See plate section.

The most likely diagnosis is:

A acne vulgaris
B erysipelas
C gingivostomatitis
D impetigo contagiosa
E rosacea

5.51 A 52-year-old woman presented with increasing tiredness and irritability and sweating that was worse at night. Her husband had complained that she had a decreased libido and was rather more forgetful. Recently she had been experiencing headaches and dizziness. She had a normal appetite and her weight had increased. She smoked 15 cigarettes per day. She did not drink alcohol or take any medication. There were no abnormal findings on examination. The next most appropriate test would be:

A 24-hour ECG
B CT head
C serum gonadotrophins
D serum prolactin
E thyroid function tests

5.52 A 55-year-old Nepalese man presented with abdominal pain. Unfortunately he spoke no English, having just arrived 2 days ago from his native Nepal. He was claiming political asylum.

On examination his temperature was 37.2°C, pulse 100 regular and blood pressure 120/70. His JVP was not elevated, heart sounds were normal and chest was clear. He had generalised abdominal tenderness but no distension. Rectal examination was normal.

Bloods				
	Hb	13.5	WCC	4.8
	Platelets	160	INR	1.4
	Na	140	K	4.2
	Urea	5.1	Creatinine	95
	Bilirubin	30	Albumin	33
	Protein	64	ALT	2400
	ALP	240	GGT	150
	Amylase	80	Glucose	4.5

Hepatitis A, B, C serology	Negative
Malaria films	Negative
Blood cultures	No growth
Chest X-ray	Normal
Abdominal ultrasound	No abnormality found in liver, gallbladder, spleen, kidneys Normal portal vein flow

Two days later, he became very drowsy with a distended abdomen and developed oliguria.

Bloods	Bilirubin	50	Albumin	27
	Protein	58	ALT	3000
	ALP	290	GGT	190
	INR	2.0	Glucose	4.0

The next most appropriate test would be:

A dengue fever serology
B hepatitis E serology
C HIV test
D paracetamol level
E yellow fever serology

5.53 A 28-year-old man was referred with difficult to control hypertension. His general practitioner had tried bendroflumethiazide (bendrofluazide) and amlodipine without success. The patient also complained of palpitations, feeling sweaty and a swelling in his neck that appeared to be getting bigger. Two years ago renal stones were diagnosed and since then had been told to drink plenty of fluids.

On examination he was an anxious young man. He had an obvious goitre but was clinically euthyroid. His pulse was 90 regular and blood pressure 170/86. His JVP was not elevated and heart sounds were normal. His chest was clear and there were no abnormal findings on abdominal examination.

Bloods	Calcium	2.75	Phosphate	0.65
	Albumin	38	PTH	1.9
	TSH	1.5	Free T$_4$	22
	Calcitonin	50		

| **24-hour urinary adrenaline (epinephrine)** | 330 |
| **24-hour urinary noradrenaline (norepinephrine)** | 750 |

The most likely diagnosis is:

A APS 1
B APS 2
C MEN 1 syndrome
D MEN 2A syndrome
E MEN 2B syndrome

5.54 A 45-year-old man presented with gross ascites. A diagnostic tap was performed on the fluid:

Serum albumin   28

Ascitic fluid albumin 26

These results would be most consistent with:

A intrabdominal malignancy with peritoneal seeding
B large bowel obstruction
C nephrotic syndrome
D portal vein thrombosis
E tuberculous peritonitis

5.55 A 19-year-old man was referred because of a 3-day history of increased thirst and polyuria. Random blood glucose was 15.8. He had no other symptoms. He had no other medical problems and was on no medication. He did not drink alcohol or smoke.
    On examination his temperature was 37.0°C, pulse 78 regular and blood pressure 115/78. The rest of the physical examination was normal. His body mass index was 23.2.

Arterial blood gases on air	pH	7.34	PCO_2	3.8
Arterial blood gases on air	PO_2	12.7	Bicarbonate	23.1
	Base excess	0.5		
Urinanalysis	Glucose 2+, ketones 1+			

The best management plan for this patient would be:

A acarbose
B diabetic diet
C gliclazide
D insulin
E metformin

5.56 A 30-year-old man was referred with ankle and facial swelling and lethargy, with proteinuria on urinary analysis. He had no previous medical history and was on no medication.
    On examination his face was puffy. He was apyrexial, pulse 88 regular and blood pressure 160/98. His JVP was not elevated and chest and heart sounds were normal. His abdomen was soft and non-tender. He had pitting oedema up to his thighs.

Bloods	Hb	13.7	WCC	4.8
	Platelets	190	INR	1.0
	Na	138	K	4.7
	Urea	12.9	Creatinine	160
	Protein	54	Albumin	25
	LDL cholesterol	8.9		

24-hour urinary protein collection   14.8 g/L

Renal biopsy   Focal segmental glomerulosclerosis

Which **ONE** of the following statements about his management is true?

A First line treatment of his oedema should be with spironolactone
B He is likely to go into and stay in remission with prednisolone
C He should be anticoagulated if his albumin drops below 25
D He would benefit from a low protein diet
E His blood pressure should be treated with bendroflumethiazide (bendrofluazide)

5.57 A 32-year-old woman presented to Accident & Emergency with pyrexia and splenomegaly. Two weeks ago she returned from holiday in West Africa (Figure 5.57). See plate section.

The organism seen in the film is:

A *Plasmodium falciparum*
B *Loa loa*
C *Leishmania donovani*
D *Trypanosoma brucei gambiense*
E *Schistosoma haematobium*

5.58 A 15-year-old boy was referred for an EEG because of fits associated with loss of consciousness. He was on no medication. While he was having another attack an EEG was performed. His EEG showed the following trace with 3 Hz spikes:

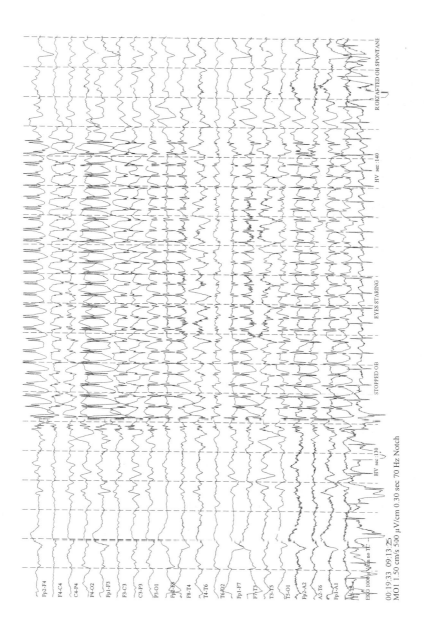

The most likely diagnosis is:

A absence seizures
B complex partial seizures
C Creutzfeldt–Jakob disease
D subacute sclerosing panencephalitis
E tonic-clonic seizures

5.59 A 37-year-old HIV-positive man was referred because of difficulty swallowing. He was not on any medication and had no other medical problems. He did not smoke or drink alcohol. Apart from oro-pharyngeal candidiasis the rest of the physical examination was normal.

Bloods   Hb   12.4   WCC   3.9

             Platelets 150

CD4   450

Viral load 16,000

The immediate treatment of choice for this patient is:

A intravenous aciclovir
B intravenous amphotericin
C intravenous ganciclovir
D oral fluconazole
E oral nystatin

5.60 A 62-year-old man was admitted with unstable angina and shortness of breath. He was treated with aspirin, diltiazem, furosemide (frusemide), glyceryl trinitrate infusion, intravenous heparin, and simvastatin. As chest pain continued coronary angiography was undertaken. This showed 75% occlusion of the left anterior descending artery and he was treated with a coronary stent. Two days later he complained of painful, discoloured toes. His renal function was noted to have deteriorated. Prior to the procedure his creatinine was 120.

On examination there were no splinter haemorrhages in his finger-nails. His temperature was 37.6°C, pulse 110 regular and blood pressure 150/90. His JVP was not elevated and chest and heart sounds were normal. Abdominal examination was normal. Toes from both feet were blue and mottled. Foot pulses and sensation were normal.

Bloods	Hb	13.8	WCC	8.9
	Neutrophils	5.8	Lymphocytes	2.1
	Eosinophils	1.0	Platelets	200
	Na	139	K	4.0
	Urea	13.8	Creatinine	250

Urinanalysis Protein 2+, blood 1+, WCC 2+, no red cell casts, eosinophils on microscopy

Chest X-ray Normal

The most likely diagnosis is:

A acute interstitial nephritis secondary to aspirin
B acute vasculitis
C cholesterol embolus
D contrast-induced nephropathy
E overdiuresis with furosemide (frusemide)

Paper 5

Answers

5.1 **D**** This patient has a history suggesting an acute coronary event but no ECG evidence. Blood tests could confirm the diagnosis and would be important for determining future prognosis. Serum LDH peaks at 72 hours and lasts for 7–10 days. Creatinine kinase peaks at 24 hours but normalizes by 48–96 hours. It may give a false-positive result in patients with chronic renal failure. Serum troponins would be most appropriate at this stage in this patient. An echocardiogram may show new wall-motion abnormalities but in the absence of a new murmur will not affect management in the present scenario. New onset left bundle branch block with a history suggestive of MI is an indication to thrombolyse.

5.2 **C**** The PR interval is getting progressively longer until after the third QRS complex the P wave is not followed by a QRS complex. This is characteristic of Wenckebach second degree AV block.

5.3 **E**** This patient presents with an oculogyric crisis, a form of drug-induced dystonia. Dopamine antagonists are well known to cause such effects. Prochlorperazine will make it worse. The correct treatment is procyclidine or benzatropine.

5.4 **A**** The patient has symptoms of headache, meningitis and fever consistent with Lyme disease. The rash is caused by the spirochaete bacterium *Borrelia burgdorferi* and starts off as an inflamed red papule, which then develops into a red, oedematous plaque with central livid regression. It may remain for many months. Erythema marginatum is associated with rheumatic fever, has a predilection for the trunk and is transient in nature. Erythema gyratum repens is a figurate erythema that is a paraneoplastic syndrome.

5.5 **A**** The patient has hypertriglyceridaemia but he is also diabetic. Before starting drug treatment this patient should try to lose weight, start a diabetic diet and reduce his alcohol intake. Metformin may be started before antilipid treatment as he is overweight and diabetic. The treatment of choice is a fibrate like gemfibrozil or bezafibrate if the triglyceride level is persistently greater than 10.

5.6 **E**** The study is flawed by the way patients were randomised. Tossing a coin is not a true randomisation procedure because, although the outcome is either 'heads' or 'tails', there may still be a disproportionate number in one group. A better method would involve a random number generator where each subject was given a number that, once chosen, would then allocate the subject to a particular treatment arm.

5.7 **A**** This patient is complaining of biliary colic. An abdominal ultrasound would readily detect gallstones and also detect whether the common bile duct was dilated.

5.8 **E**** This is a sequestration crisis as there is sudden drop in haemoglobin with the red blood cells being trapped in the liver, which enlarges rapidly; in a younger child this may also occur in the spleen. These can occur repeatedly, over a very short period of time and may be life-threatening. Treatment involves transfusion, hydration, preventing hypoxia, opioid analgesia and possibly splenectomy if there is splenic sequestration. Chest syndrome is characterised by pleuritic chest pain, anoxia and anaemia from pulmonary vessel blockage. Aplastic crises can occur secondary to parvovirus infection and result in a rapid fall in haemoglobin levels without other clinical findings; the reticulocyte count is low, which differentiates it from haemolytic crises, where there is marked haemolysis complicating a painful/infarctive crisis. Infarctive crises are characterised by bone pain.

5.9 **E**** The slide shows a lymph node, which stains blue. The large pink lesion represents granuloma, which would be consistent with sarcoidosis. If this were lymphoma the whole slide would appear blue with lymphoid cells. Lung carcinoma consists of large pleomorphic cells with big nucleoli. Reactive lymphadenopathy is associated with an exaggerated normal architecture with large germinal centres. Tuberculous granulomas show caseation.

5.10 **B**** This patient is HBsAg-positive and anti-HBc-positive meaning that she has been exposed to hepatitis B. As she is IgM-HBc negative this would suggest that she does not have acute hepatitis B. HBeAg and HBV DNA are indicators of active replication; in this case she is not actively replicating and she is anti-Hbe-positive. Very rarely some patients can have a precore mutation whereby they are still replicating but are HBeAg-negative. Patients who are immune or vaccinated to hepatitis B will be HBsAg-negative and anti-HBs positive.

5.11 **B***** This woman has myasthenia gravis (see **4.11**), which can be confirmed by finding anti-acetylcholine receptor antibodies, single-muscle fibre electro-myography or an edrophonium/tensilon test. Edrophonium is a short acting anticholinesterase, which will cause an improvement in muscle weakness and fatiguability if patients have myasthenia gravis.

5.12 **B*** This patient has malignant hypertensive retinopathy. There is swelling of the optic disc with definite blurring of the disc margin, severely attenuated arteries, cotton wool spots, scattered flame-shaped haemorrhages, dilated tortuous veins and a partial macular star. The fundus looks tessellated, which is a normal variant. Note this cannot be defined as papilloedema because papilloedema is bilateral optic disc swelling due to raised intraocular pressure only and not secondary to malignant hypertension.

5.13 **C**** A young man presents to casualty with status asthmaticus. He has features of life- threatening asthma: inability to perform peak flow; unable to complete sentences; using accessory muscles of respiration; hypotension; respiratory rate >30 breaths/min; acidosis and increasing PCO_2. He has already had nebulised salbutamol and 200 mg of intravenous hydrocortisone, with little improvement in his clinical state. All of the management steps would help his current situation and he may well need to be ventilated very soon if there is no further improvement or he becomes more tired. Intravenous magnesium has been shown to improve severe asthma. In this case there is no evidence of chest infection/pneumonia so antibiotics would not be indicated.

BTS/SIGN. British Guideline on the Management of Asthma. Thorax. Feb 2003: 58 Supp I.

5.14 **B**** This woman has thickened skin, Raynaud's phenomenon, oesophageal dysmotility symptoms and telangiectasia. All of these features, along with positive anticentromere antibodies, would be consistent with CREST syndrome, although calcinosis is absent. The upper gastrointestinal haemorrhage is due to bleeding from the gastric telangiectasia. This is unlikely to be systemic sclerosis because she has negative anti-SCL antibodies, normal renal function and skin involvement limited to the hands. Amyloidosis can affect the gastrointestinal system and can cause haemorrhage but is usually secondary to another chronic illness like rheumatoid arthritis if it is not associated with myeloma. Hereditary haemorrhagic telangiectasia is not associated with Raynaud's phenomenon or arthralgia. Raynaud's phenomenon may be the initial symptom of CREST syndrome.

5.15 **A***** Barrett's oesophagus is defined as metaplastic change in the squamous epithelial lining of the oesophagus. With chronic reflux this changes to a more reddish, gastric columnar epithelial lining. It produces no symptoms but may lead to adenocarcinoma.

5.16 **D**** The CT scan shows a chronic left subdural haematoma. It is due to tearing of the bridging veins and blood collects between the dura and the arachnoid. The lesion follows the shape of the brain to display a more 'semi-circular' appearance. Compare and contrast this with 1.17.

5.17 **E**** This patient has a ring-enhancing lesion on his CT head. The differential diagnosis in a patient with HIV would be toxoplasmosis, lymphoma or abscess. The most sensible treatment option, after taking all appropriate cultures, would be to treat as though he had cerebral toxoplasmosis. There is no midline shift and therefore no need to start steroids.

5.18 C** The fixed, split second heart sound is the hallmark of atrial septal defect. There may be a systolic murmur, heard loudest in the pulmonary area because of increased flow across the pulmonary valve. Patients may present with cyanosis, clubbing and a loud second heart sound when pulmonary hypertension and Eisenmenger's complex develop. On the ECG there may be incomplete or complete right bundle branch block. If there is a secundum lesion with a patent fossa ovalis then there is right axis deviation. With ostium primum lesions, which occur just above the atrioventricular valves, there is left axis deviation.

5.19 D** This patient presents with signs and symptoms of Wallenberg's syndrome or lateral medullary syndrome. The vessel that is usually occluded is likely to be the posterior inferior cerebellar artery, a branch of the vertebral artery. The clinical effects are ipsilateral V, VI, VII and VIII cranial nerve lesions, ipsilateral bulbar palsy, ipsilateral Horner's syndrome and ipsilateral cerebellar lesion. The jerking nystagmus on turning the head may make the patient complain of diplopia. Damage to the lateral spinothalamic and, sometimes, pyramidal tracts will cause contralateral hemianaesthesiae and upper motor neurone signs in the arm and leg.

5.20 D** This patient has tophi, which appear as nodular structures, usually around joints, especially in the foot, and ear lobes. If the overlying skin is eroded they may discharge a whitish, crumbling mass, which if analysed microscopically will often show sodium urate needles. Tophi may occur after an acute attack of gout and may be painless. Heberden's nodes affect the distal interphalangeal joints but the joint per se does not look inflamed. Rheumatoid nodules hardly ever affect the distal interphalangeal joints.

5.21 A** The answer is normal bone mass as both her T score and Z score are above –1. For an explanation of how to interpret DEXA scan results see 1.7.

5.22 D* This pregnant patient has fever, low platelet count with associated bruising, impaired renal function, neurological changes and evidence of micro-angiopathic haemolytic anaemia, which are all features of thrombotic thrombocytopenic purpura. This can be differentiated from disseminated intravascular coagulopathy because there is normal clotting. Similarly, acute fatty liver of pregnancy and HELLP syndrome would be associated with marked derangement of liver function tests. HELLP is associated with pre-eclampsia, which is characterised by hypertension, proteinuria and oedema. Toxic shock syndrome is produced by toxin producing Gram-positive bacteria and is associated with temperature >38.9°, macular rash, abdominal pain and diarrhoea, and is more likely in menstruating females using highly absorbent tampons.

5.23 C** The specificity is the proportion of patients who do not have the disease, which the test excludes as not having the condition.

	Lung cancer +	Lung cancer −	
CT +	60 (a)	25 (b)	85
CT −	80 (c)	335 (d)	415
	140	360	500

Specificity = d/d+b = 335/360 = 0.93%

5.24 C** Middle-aged woman with history of ascites, weakness and pruritis with cholestatic liver picture is very suggestive of primary biliary cirrhosis. In most cases of pruritis there is release of histamine and so chlorpheniramine, an anti-histamine, is very useful. However, in primary biliary cirrhosis, the main problem is cholestasis and so a bile acid sequestrant such as cholestyramine is used. The other treatment for primary biliary cirrhosis is urso deoxycholic acid (UDCA). Steroids and azathioprine are used in autoimmune hepatitis. Penicillamine is used to treat Wilson's disease.

5.25 E** A boy presents with bruising, pyrexia, lymphadenopathy and spleno-megaly. Full blood count shows low platelet count, leucopenia and normal haemoglobin. All these features would be consistent with infectious mono-nucleosis or glandular fever. It must always be a differential diagnosis for cervical lymphadenopathy. Acute myeloid leukaemia can be associated with gum hypertrophy. The fact that there are no blasts on the film goes against this being acute leukaemia. Although not always the case, infectious mono-nucleosis can be associated with atypical lymphocytes on the blood film.

5.26 A** In the centre of the slide is a capillary with infected endothelial cells. Cytomegalovirus is characterised by bloated endothelial cells with inclusion bodies and occasional nuclear 'owl's eye inclusions'. With TB, there would be caseating granulomas. With *M. avium intracellulare* there would be more cells out in the periphery with clear cytoplasm. Kaposi's sarcoma is associated with spindle cells with red cells in between.

5.27 E** Syringomyelia results from a longitudinal cystic cavity that develops within the spinal cord and which may extend over a number of segments or even into the medulla (syringobulbia). The clinical features are those of a myelopathy or disease affecting the spinal cord. At the level of the syrinx, the involvement of the anterior horn cells causes a lower motor neurone lesion that results in wasting of the upper limb muscles and decreased tone and reflexes. For some unknown reason fasciculation is uncommon. The dissociated sensory loss is due to involvement of the lateral spinothalamic tract but sparing of the dorsal columns. Below the level of the syrinx there can be involvement of the pyramidal tracts, causing a spastic paraparesis. The Horner's syndrome is due to involvement of the cervical sympathetic nerves. A Pancoast's tumour could also produce wasting of the small muscles of the hand due to involvement of the lower brachial plexus and Horner's syndrome, but would not cause bilateral lower limb signs or kyphoscoliosis.

Cervical myelopathy can produce the spastic paraparesis and wasting of the small muscles of the hand but not the Horner's syndrome. HSMN can present as wasting of the small muscles of the hand but could not explain the dissociated sensory loss and pyramidal signs.

5.28 B** This patient with COPD has a normal PO_2 but evidence of uncompensated respiratory acidosis. Her drowsiness may be due to carbon dioxide narcosis. She may have carbon dioxide retention, which could get worse on increasing her oxygen concentration. The safest option would be to reduce the oxygen concentration to see if there is an improvement in her acidosis. If there is worsening acidosis and the PCO_2 remains elevated then there should be serious consideration for invasive ventilation.

5.29 C* Presentation with peripheral neuropathy, vasculitic rash, arthralgia, mild renal impairment and a history of hepatitis B infection are features that would be consistent with polyarteritis nodosa. This is a vasculitis of small and medium-sized blood vessels. When associated with hepatitis B infection, patients tend to be e antigen and HBV DNA positive but ANCA antibodies are negative. Unlike cryoglobulinaemia there are normal complement levels. Microscopic polyangiitis is more associated with alveolar haemorrhage, not associated with hepatitis B, and p-ANCA is positive in 50–80% of cases.

5.30 D* *M. marinum* can produce 'fish tank granulomas', which are bluish-red inflammatory nodules that occur at the sites of injury and track up the arm or leg. They can ulcerate but are not infectious.

5.31 C** The X-ray shows enlargement of the sella turcica and erosion of the dorsum sella. This would be consistent with a hypophyseal/pituitary tumour.

5.32 E*** This patient has oesophageal varices. On endoscopy they will appear as round projections arranged in columns. With a barium swallow the filling defects reflect their round shape. Oesophageal candidiasis appears as straight columns (see **2.33**).

5.33 A* This patient has Fallot's tetralogy and almost certainly had a Blalock–Taussig shunt (brachial to pulmonary artery anastomosis) as an infant. The clinical features are: pulmonary stenosis, ventricular septal defect (with right-to-left shunt), right ventricular hypertrophy and overriding aorta. Squatting improves symptoms because it increases systemic vascular resistance and so reduces the amount of blood returning to the heart and hence through the right-to-left shunt. This can lead to pooling of blood in the legs. Eisenmenger's syndrome is when there is reversal of flow in conditions that produce left-to-right shunts. β-Blockers reduce right ventricular outflow obstruction.

5.34 E* The cardiac monitor shows a trace that resembles atrial fibrillation; however, in the context of a patient with no pulse, this is pulseless electrical activity or electromechanical dissociation. Cardiopulmonary resuscitation should be attempted in patients who do not have VF/VT; in this case, chest compressions followed by 1 mg adrenaline (epinephrine) intravenously after every 3 minutes. In the meantime, aim to treat the cause; in this case it is likely to be hypovolaemic shock.

5.35 D** This patient has a photosensitive dermatitis affecting the back of the neck. Amiodarone is associated with photosensitivity, digoxin is not.

5.36 B** This patient could possibly have a cold nodule that may be malignant. The only way to be sure is to do a fine needle aspiration. Ultrasound would reveal whether the nodule was cystic or not. Isotope scanning would reveal whether it is a hot or cold nodule, depending on whether it takes up tracer. A significant proportion of cold nodules are malignant and hence fine needle aspiration is mandatory.

5.37 E** This test fits most of the criteria for a screening test: easy to administer, high sensitivity and specificity, inexpensive, not harmful to patients and the disease is not too rare. The only problem is that CJD is incurable and the screening test can only be used after the patient has presented with the clinical disease. Screening tests ideally should detect the disease before clinical problems develop so that future management can be altered.

5.38 A** A middle-aged man presents with acute pancreatitis. He is on a number of drugs which could have caused this, including steroids, mesalazine and azathioprine. Hypercalcaemia is another cause of acute pancreatitis. With time, saponification occurs, which results in hypocalcaemia. Treatment is usually conservative because there is a very high mortality if operations are undertaken in the first 2 weeks. ERCP may be a cause of pancreatitis but if the condition is due to gallstones then endoscopic pancreatic duct decompression may be beneficial. Alcohol is the usual cause of acute pancreatitis. The serum amylase usually confirms the diagnosis of pancreatitis but adds nothing to predicting a patient's prognosis. For that, Ranson's criteria are used, taking measurements at admission (age > 55 years; WCC > 15; glucose > 10; LDH > 600 and AST > 60) and at 48 hours (haematocrit drop > 10%; urea > 16; PO_2 < 8; calcium < 2; albumin < 32 and base excess > −4).

5.39 E** Bulbar palsy is a syndrome of lower motor neurone paralysis that affects the muscles innervated by the cranial nerves that originate in the medulla/bulb. Unlike bulbar palsy, pseudobulbar palsy is an upper motor neurone lesion and does not originate in the brainstem. It affects the corticobulbar system above the brainstem bilaterally to produce similar clinical features. Dysarthria and dysphagia are common to both but the palate and pharynx are hyperactive in pseudobulbar palsy. Bulbar palsy speech has a more nasal twang and the tongue is flaccid and fasciculating. Jugular foramen syndrome affects IX, X and XI cranial nerves, and presents with palatal paralysis, uvula drawn up to the contralateral side, absent gag reflex and weakness and wasting of sternocleidomastoid. Cerebellopontine angle lesions involve V, VI, VII, VIII and cerebellum to produce ipsilateral loss of corneal reflex, VI and VII nerve palsies, perceptive deafness and cerebellar impairment. Medial medullary syndrome results in ipsilateral paresis of the tongue, contralateral hemiplegia and contralateral loss of joint position and vibration sense.

5.40 C* The normal flow–volume should have a triangular expiratory loop (above the x-axis) and a semicircular inspiratory loop (below the x-axis). With emphysema there is pressure dependent collapse of the airways soon after expiration occurs which results in the early drop in the expiratory limb. With chronic bronchitis and asthma, there is a normal inspiratory loop but there is a more gradual flattening of the expiratory limb (volume dependent collapse). If there is a fixed intrathoracic or extrathoracic lesion like goitre or lymph nodes then there is flattening of both inspiratory and expiratory limbs.

5.41 D** This young man presents with urethritis, conjunctivitis and arthritis, which may have followed a urogenital infection by *Chlamydia trachomatis*. The heel pain and thickening of the Achilles' tendon would be consistent with enthesitis, which is inflammation of the ligaments and tendons that is characteristic of 'reactive arthritides'. Gonococcal arthritis does not cause enthesitis or conjunctivitis and is associated with a migratory arthritis. Behçet's syndrome is associated with orogenital ulceration, arthritis and eye symptoms but not enthesitis, and usually presents with skin lesions.

5.42 B** The photograph shows a reddish-brown discoloration of the patient's ear. The disease affects the cartilaginous pinna, with sparing of the inferior soft lobules. With progressive dissolution of the cartilage the ear becomes floppy ('cauliflower ear'). The nasal cartilage can also be affected, resulting in a 'saddle-shaped' deformity.

5.43 E* There is blood in the left Sylvian fissure consistent with a subarachnoid haemorrhage. Compare both sides of the CT head scan. On the right there appears to be a low attenuation (black) line, whereas on the left this line is high attenuation (white).

5.44 E** This patient has the rash and symptoms of Henoch–Schönlein purpura. HSP is a type of vasculitis and type III hypersensitivity. It may develop post-viral or poststreptococcal infection and is associated with headache, malaise, abdominal pain, arthralgia, haematuria and possibly glomerulonephritis. The rash consists of sharply demarcated pink or red haemorrhagic patches, mainly on the lower limbs and buttocks. As it is a vasculitis there is no thrombocytopenia. Skin biopsy would show deposits of IgA about the dermal vessels. There is no effective treatment.

5.45 E*** This patient has Conn's syndrome (see **3.58**). As she is most likely to have an aldosteronone-secreting adenoma, the best drug would be an aldosterone antagonist: spironolactone. The definitive treatment would be to localise the tumour and perform an adrenalectomy.

5.46 B** This patient has a history and examination findings suggestive of acute colitis. Toxic megacolon needs to be excluded. The most appropriate investigation should be a plain abdominal X-ray. The other tests can be performed at a later date if necessary.

5.47 D* Status epilepticus is a medical emergency and should be managed aggressively as there is a risk of permanent nerurological damage, coma and death. Pyrexia and urine that shows blood but not haemoglobin is a possible indicator that this patient may have rhabdomyolysis. The main aim of treatment is to abolish the fits using a benzodiazepine. This can be with either diazepam or lorazepam. If this should fail to control them, intravenous phenytoin should be administered. Phenobarbital can also be given but by this stage an anaesthetist ought to be assessing the patient for ventilation. Patients who continue to fit should be moved to a place where they will not harm themselves, but only when their fits have stopped; no attempt should be made to move them while they are fitting.

5.48 C** Certain signs and symptoms suggest that low back pain is not due to a mechanical, inflammatory or soft tissue cause. These include the pain that does not respond to changes in position; pain associated with fever, rigors and weight loss; bilateral pain that is progressive; and abnormal neurological signs.

5.49 E*** There is loss of the haustral folds and superficial ulceration from the rectum in continuity to the mid-transverse colon. This would be consistent with ulcerative colitis rather than the discontinuous lesions of Crohn's colitis or the predominant splenic flexure location of ischaemic colitis.

5.50 E** Rosacea is a disease characterised by papules and pustules on the central face, against a livid erythematous background with telangiectasia, and is exacerbated by sunlight. Acne vulgaris would be an unusual presentation so late in adulthood; it is characterised by pustules and comedones.

5.51 C** This patient presents with all the features of a woman going through the menopause. Other symptoms include amenorrhoea, depression, arthralgia and hot flushes. Such patients would be expected to have a high FSH and high LH.

5.52 **D*** A patient presents with acute liver failure. There is a possibility he may have a viral haemorrhagic fever, although he would be expected to be more jaundiced and show signs of bleeding. Hepatitis E has an incubation period of 3–9 weeks so it is possible that he may have been harbouring this virus. However, the test is only carried out in specialist centres where there is a high index of suspicion. HIV can cause very deranged liver function tests but testing for this should not be considered a first-line investigation. Paracetamol overdose is very common and must be excluded along with salicylate overdose in any patient with unexplained deranged liver function tests.

5.53 **D*** The cause of this patient's hypertension is phaeochromocytoma, as shown by the high urinary catecholamines and the failure to respond to thiazide diuretics and calcium antagonists (see **1.53**). He also has hyperparathyroidism and this has caused renal calculi in the past. The goitre and high calcitonin level are associated with medullary carcinoma of the thyroid. These are all associated with MEN 2A syndromes. MEN 2B syndromes are associated with hyperplasia or neoplastic transformation of the thyroid parafollicular cells and adrenal medulla with concomitant development of mucosal neuromas and possibly a Marfanoid appearance.

5.54 **D*** The serum–ascites albumin gradient gives an indication of whether a patient has portal hypertension or not. If $albumin_{serum} - albumin_{ascites} \geq 1.1$ then the patient has portal hypertension. Causes of portal hypertension include: cirrhosis; portal vein thrombosis; Budd–Chiari syndrome; venoocclusive disease; fatty liver of pregnancy and myxoedema. All the other causes in the question are associated with a low gradient.

5.55 **D**** This young patient with new onset diabetes is likely to be insulin dependent diabetic. At the moment he is becoming symptomatic of diabetes and unless he is started on insulin very soon he will develop ketoacidosis.

5.56 **C**** This patient has nephrotic syndrome secondary to FSGS. FSGS is a type of glomerulonephritis characterised by focal mesangial collapse of some gloerumeruli and segmental scarring in part of the glomerular capillary tufts. Fifty per cent of patients with heavy proteinuria go on to develop end-stage renal failure. Raised blood pressure should be treated with ACE inhibitors and/or angiotensin II antagonists because these drugs have been shown to reduce glomerular causes of proteinuria. Hyperlipidaemia should be treated with statins; and oedema should be treated with loop diuretics, not spironolactone. Another complication of nephrotic syndrome is an increased thrombotic tendency, which is believed to be due to a combination of a loss of anticoagulants and increased production of procoagulants. An albumin <25 is arbitrarily set as the point at which to start anticoagulation. Low protein diet is controversial as it may decrease the protein-losing state but may make the hypoalbuminaemia worse. Unlike minimal change glomerulonephritis or membranous nephropathy, FSGS patients often fail to remain in remission with steroids.

5.57 D* The blood film shows the characteristic 'S-shaped' trypomastigotes between blood cells. African trypanosomiasis or sleeping sickness is a disease caused by protozoa carried by tsetse flies. There are two types: *T. brucei gambiense* (West Africa) and *rhodesiense* (East Africa).

5.58 A* EEGs are difficult to interpret but absence seizures are associated with a characteristic waveform. The discharges appear and discharge suddenly but have a regular 3 spike per second frequency. CJD and subacute sclerosing panencephalitis also have characteristic waveforms but are a lot slower, lasting 1 second and 4–14 seconds respectively. Complex partial seizures are characterised by spikes followed by slow waves.

5.59 D*** This patient has oropharyngeal candidiasis and so it would be safe to presume that he has oesophageal candidiasis as the cause of his symptoms. The correct treatment is oral fluconazole. Only if his symptoms persist after treatment would upper GI endoscopy be indicated to look for another cause.

5.60 C* This patient has developed a cholesterol embolus, as suggested by the discoloration of the toes due to small vessel infarction, mild fever and eosinophilia and eosoinophiluria. Such complications can occur after invasive procedures such as angioplasty. Acute interstitial nephritis can also cause fever and eosinophilia but does not give toe discoloration. Contrast-induced nephropathy and overdiuresis with furosemide (frusemide) are not associated with eosinophilia. Acute vasculitis would be unlikely, given the time frame and lack of active urinary sediment.

Questions

6.1 A 49-year-old man was admitted with an inferior MI. He was treated with streptokinase and appeared to make a good recovery, becoming pain free. He had no previous medical history. He was a heavy smoker. Twelve hours later he became acutely unwell, feeling cold, clammy and sweating. He had no shortness of breath or palpitations but had a recurrence of his chest pain.

On examination he was unwell and in pain. His temperature was 35.9°C, pulse 110 regular and blood pressure 80/45. His JVP was elevated to +8 cm but his heart sounds were normal and there were no murmurs or added sounds. His chest was clear and his abdomen soft and non-tender.

Bloods				
	Hb	14.2	WCC	12.4
	Platelets	234	INR	1.1
	Na	138	K	4.8
	Urea	4.7	Creatinine	78
	Magnesium	0.90	Calcium	2.23
	Amylase	24	Albumin	38
	Protein	65	Bilirubin	12
	ALT	25	ALP	75

Chest X-ray	Normal
ECG	ST elevation in II, III and aVF
	ST depression in V_{1-3}
	Normal sinus rhythm

Arterial blood gases on air	pH	7.39	PCO_2	3.52
	PO_2	13.8	Bicarbonate	22.8
	Base excess	1.0		

The most likely complication this patient has suffered is:

A cardiac tamponade
B pulmonary embolism
C right ventricular infarction
D rupture of the interventricular septum
E rupture of the papillary muscles

6.2 A 53-year-old woman was admitted with central crushing chest pain while walking to work.

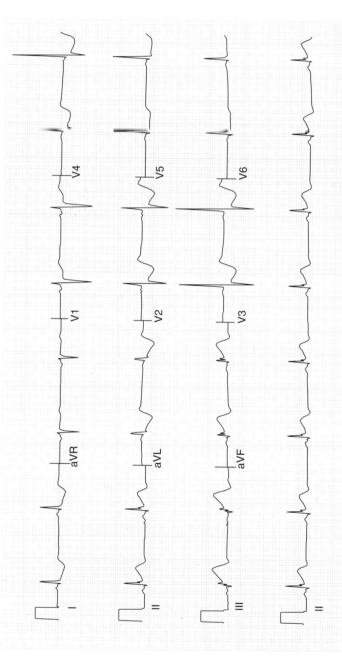

Her ECG shows:

A anterior MI
B anterolateral MI
C inferior MI
D inferolateral MI
E inferoposterior MI

6.3 A 16-year-old girl was brought to Accident & Emergency in a state of collapse. She had been at a nightclub and her friends thought she might have taken something there. Normally she was fit and well and not on any medication.

On examination she was drowsy but responded to command. She was disorientated in time and place. Her temperature was 40.6°C, pulse 120 regular and blood pressure 195/114. Her JVP was not elevated and heart sounds were normal. Her chest was clear. Abdominal examination was normal. She was uncooperative on neurological examination but her pupils were dilated and her plantars were flexor. She only passed 40 mL of urine over the preceding 4 hours.

Bloods	Hb	10.8	WCC	5.4
	Platelets	100	INR	1.4
	Na	130	K	6.9
	Urea	22.3	Creatinine	328
	Protein	64	Albumin	37
	Bilirubin	15	ALT	350
	ALP	140	Calcium	1.81
	Phosphate	1.82		

Chest X-ray	Normal			
Arterial blood gases on air	pH	7.29	PCO_2	2.9
	PO_2	12.5	Bicarbonate	12.3
	Base excess	−13.1		

Which **ONE** of the following statements concerning this patient's condition is **FALSE**?

A Alkalinisation of urine with bicarbonate is indicated
B Dipstick and microscopy of her urine is likely to show blood and red blood cells.
C Hypertension should be treated with labetalol infusion
D Mannitol diuresis should be considered if oliguria persists in spite of intravenous fluid resuscitation
E She is at risk of compartment syndrome

6.4 A 58-year-old woman was referred with weight loss and anorexia. On examination she had a rash in her axilla (Figure 6.4). See plate section.

Of the following, the condition **LEAST** likely to be associated with this skin rash is:

A carcinoma of the breast
B carcinoma of the colon
C carcinoma of the kidney
D carcinoma of the pancreas
E carcinoma of the uterus

6.5 A 27-year-old woman presented with shortness of breath, tiredness and a swelling of her neck over the past 2 weeks.

Thyroid function TSH	0.4	Total T_4	200
Free T_4	15	Total T_3	2.0

The most likely explanation for these results is:

A pregnancy
B primary hyperthyroidism
C sick euthyroid syndrome
D subacute (de Quervain's) thyroiditis
E surreptitious treatment with thyroxine

6.6 Two thousand patients with multiple sclerosis were randomly allocated to treatment with β-interferon or placebo. At the end of 5 years 20 patients in the β-interferon group had severe relapse, compared with 100 of the placebo group. The absolute risk reduction (ARR) in relapse due to β-interferon is:

A 0.02
B 0.08
C 0.10
D 0.12
E 0.80

6.7 A 39-year-old man with alcoholic liver disease was admitted with jaundice and abdominal distension. He last had a drink of alcohol 24 hours ago. He was only on thiamine tablets.

   On examination he was apyrexial and very jaundiced. He was verbally abusive and, although awake, was completely disorientated. His tongue was furred and his skin turgor reduced. There were no signs of bleeding. His pulse was 72 regular and blood pressure 110/60. Respiratory examination was normal. He had moderate ascites and bilateral leg oedema up to the thighs. Rectal examination revealed dark brown faeces. After catheterisation he passed 100 mL over 6 hours.

Bloods	Hb	10.1	MCV	100.2
	WCC	9.4	Platelets	85
	INR	1.8	Na	117
	K	3.0	Urea	8.5
	Creatinine	96	Albumin	27
	Protein	54	Bilirubin	320
	ALT	145	ALP	250

Arterial blood gas on air	pH	7.30	PCO_2	4.0
	PO_2	8.6	Bicarbonate	18
	Base excess	−6.5		

Chest X-ray   Normal

The most important next step in the management of this patient would be to:

  A correct dehydration with normal saline adding potassium to each bag
  B fluid restrict to 1.5 litres per day and give intravenous furosemide (frusemide)
  C give diazepam regularly to prevent withdrawal fits
  D give lactulose
  E transfuse two units of blood as he may have bleeding varices

6.8   A 23-year-old Afro-Caribbean man was referred with sudden abdominal pain, jaundice and haematuria. He was due to go to Egypt on holiday next week and had been given malaria prophylaxis, which he had started to take 4 days ago. He had a normal appetite and no weight loss. He had no previous medical problems and was not on any medication.

     On examination he was jaundiced. His temperature was 37.0°C, pulse 100 regular and his blood pressure 100/65. Cardiovascular and respiratory examination was normal. There was generalised abdominal tenderness but no organomegaly.

Bloods	Hb	8.2	MCV	99.5
	WCC	4.7	Platelets	300
	Reticulocytes	15%	INR	1.0
	Na	135	K	4.0
	Urea	3.3	Creatinine	70
	Protein	65	Albumin	37
	Bilirubin	80	ALT	25
	ALP	80		

Blood film   Heinz bodies

Urinanalysis   Urobilinogen 2+, no bilirubin, haemoglobin 2+, blood 1+

**Direct
Coombs' test**   Negative

The most likely diagnosis is:

    A autoimmune haemolytic anaemia
    B Gilbert's syndrome
    C G6PD deficiency
    D hereditary spherocytosis
    E pyruvate kinase deficiency

6.9   A 31-year-old man with HIV was admitted with shortness of breath and cough productive of blood-streaked yellow sputum for the past 2 weeks. He had decreased appetite and loss of weight. He smoked 20 cigarettes per day but did not drink alcohol. He had no previous medical problems and was not on any medication.

    On examination his temperature was 37.9°C, pulse 100 regular and blood pressure 110/62. His JVP was not elevated and heart sounds were normal. He had decreased breath sounds on the right side.

Chest X-ray   Right hilar shadowing

Bronchoscopy was performed and washings were taken (Figure 6.9). See plate section.

The most likely diagnosis is:

    A Cytomegalovirus pneumonitis
    B Kaposi's sarcoma
    C Lymphoma
    D *Mycobacterium* TB
    E *Pneumocystis carinii* pneumonia

6.10   A 30-year-old woman was 20 weeks pregnant and was found to be HIV-positive. She was otherwise fit and well. She had no other medical problems and was on no treatment. No abnormalities were found on physical examination.

CD4   800

Viral load 12,000

Which **ONE** of the following statements concerning her management is correct?

  A As she is asymptomatic she does not need to start anti-HIV treatment
  B Normal vaginal delivery is not contraindicated
  C HIV is not a contraindication to breast feeding her baby
  D The baby must be given AZT for the first 6 weeks of life
  E Vertical transmission of HIV is greatest during the first trimester

6.11 A 55-year-old woman presented with inability to walk but she had normal use of her arms. Her problem started 2 days ago and was getting worse. Bowels and micturition were normal. Two weeks ago she had a bout of gastroenteritis but made an uneventful recovery. There was no previous medical history and she was not on any medication. She smoked 20 cigarettes per day.

On examination she was not in pain. Her pulse was 90 regular and blood pressure 130/94. Her chest was clear. There was no palpable bladder and she had normal anal tone. She was unable to stand. There was no muscle wasting or fasciculation in her legs. Tone was decreased, power was 0/5 and reflexes were absent. Pinprick sensation was reduced up to the ankle. Upper limbs and cranial nerve examination were normal.

Bloods	Hb	13.5		WCC	5.6
	Platelets	198		ESR	30
	Glucose	4.5			
CSF	Glucose	3.0		Protein	1.2
	WCC	10			

The most likely diagnosis is:

  A Guillain–Barre syndrome
  B motor neurone disease
  C multiple sclerosis
  D poliomyelitis
  E transverse myelitis

6.12 A 49-year-old woman was referred with deteriorating vision. Fundoscopy was performed and is shown below (Figure 6.12). See plate section.

The following **TWO** abnormalities shown are:

A cholesterol embolus
B cotton wool spots
C flame-shaped retinal haemorrhage
D hard exudates
E microaneurysms
F optic atrophy
G papilloedema
H preretinal (subhyaloid) haemorrhage
I retinal detachment
J vitreous haemorrhage

6.13 A 45-year-old man with known squamous cell carcinoma of the lung was admitted because of progressive weakness. Surgery was not considered an option in this patient and he was being treated only with chemotherapy. He complained of abdominal pain, nausea and loose stools but no bleeding anywhere.

On examination he was not in pain but looked cachexic. He was apyrexial, pulse 100 regular and blood pressure 130/70. He had some crackles in the right mid-zone where the tumour was. Abdominal examination was normal. He had weakness but no wasting of the quadriceps and there was normal tone, reflexes and sensation.

Bloods	Hb	9.9	WCC	3.5
	Platelets	100	Na	138
	K	2.5	Urea	3.8
	Creatinine	69	Protein	62
	Albumin	34	Bilirubin	15
	ALT	30	ALP	120
	Glucose	7.5	Calcium	2.1
	Bicarbonate	34		

Chest X-ray Solitary irregular lesion in right mid-zone

The most likely cause for his deterioration is due to:

A carcinomatous neuropathy
B ectopic ACTH secretion
C hypocalcaemia
D hypomagnesaemia secondary to cisplatin
E metastatic disease

6.14 A 48-year-old woman was referred with progressive pain in her hands and wrists, which was worse in the morning, for about 6 months. She complained that her hands hurt a lot and that they changed colour when it got cold. She also described problems with chewing and swallowing her food. She had an underactive thyroid gland but apart from thyroxine was not on any other medication. She did not smoke or drink alcohol.

On examination her pulse was 74 regular and blood pressure 134/88. Respiratory examination was normal. Her wrists and metacarpophalangeal joints were swollen and tender but the other joints were normal.

Bloods				
	Hb	13.5	WCC	3.4
	Platelets	160	Na	139
	K	4.4	Urea	5.5
	Creatinine	88	Protein	80
	Albumin	38	Bilirubin	16
	ALT	19	ALP	78
	ESR	65	CRP	120

Rheumatoid factor	1 in 160
Antinuclear antibody	1 in 80
Anti-DS DNA	Negative
Anticentromere antibody	Negative
Anti-Ro antibody	1 in 80
Anti-La antibody	1 in 40
Anti-Jo1 antibody	Negative

The most likely diagnosis is:

A mixed connective tissue disease
B Reiter's disease
C Sjögren's syndrome
D systemic lupus erythematosus
E systemic sclerosis

6.15 A 10-year-old girl was referred with temporary loss of vision. She had been deaf since birth (Figure 6.15). See plate section.

The most likely congenital infection she has is:

A cytomegalovirus
B herpes simplex virus
C rubella
D syphilis
E toxoplasmosis

6.16 A 52-year-old man was referred because of progressive shortness of breath, chronic cough and weight loss. He had smoked 15 cigarettes per day for over 30 years. Until recently he was a coal miner (Figure 6.16). (See plate section).

The likely interpretation of the radiological abnormality is:

    A Caplan's syndrome
    B cor pulmonale
    C cryptogenic fibrosing alveolitis
    D mesothelioma
    E metastatic thyroid carcinoma

6.17 A 14-year-old boy presented to Accident & Emergency very unwell. While riding his bicycle he fell and sustained a cut to his left thigh. He was able to walk and the bleeding was not heavy but his leg was now very swollen and tender.

    On examination he was in a lot of pain. His temperature was 38.2°C, pulse 110 regular and blood pressure 90/55. He had decreased range of movements of his left lower limb due to pain, although sensation and peripheral pulses were normal (Figure 6.17). See plate section.

The most likely organism to have caused his symptoms is:

    A *Clostridium botulinum*
    B *Clostridium septicum*
    C *Clostridium tetani*
    D *Staphyloccus aureus*
    E *Streptococcus pyogenes*

6.18 A 22-year-old man collapsed while playing squash. This was the third time he had had such an episode while playing sports. There was no chest pain or shortness of breath. He did not smoke or drink and was not on any medication. His father died suddenly at the age of 35.

    On examination he looked well. His pulse was 94 regular and blood pressure 122/88. The JVP was not elevated but there was a thrusting apex beat. There was an ejection systolic murmur that did not radiate to the carotids. Respiratory and central nervous system examinations were normal.

ECG   Q waves in I, aVL, V_{5-6}

            T wave inversion I, aVL, V_{5-6}

            Voltage criteria for left ventricular hypertrophy

The drug treatment of choice for this patient is:

A atenolol
B digoxin
C enalapril
D furosemide (frusemide)
E isosorbide mononitrate

6.19 A 69-year-old man with a family history of ischaemic heart disease and strokes was admitted with progressive shortness of breath, but no chest pain. He did not smoke or drink alcohol. His only medication was aspirin.

On examination his temperature was 37.0°C, pulse 80 regular and blood pressure 120/79. His JVP was not elevated and heart sounds were normal. His chest was clear. Blood tests were normal.

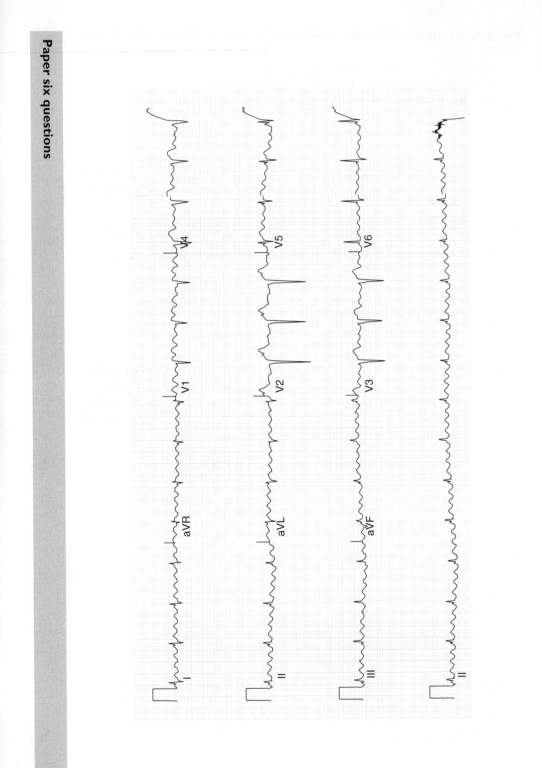

Which **ONE** of the following statements concerning management of this patient is true?

    A Adenosine often terminates this condition
    B Anticoagulation should be considered in this patient
    C Flecainide would be contraindicated
    D A permanent pacemaker should be inserted
    E Immediate DC cardioversion is the treatment of choice

6.20 A 35-year-old man was referred with a lesion on his right knee. He had similar lesions on his other knee and on both buttocks (Figure 6.20). See plate section.

Which **ONE** of the following statements concerning this patient is **FALSE**?

    A He is likely to have a normal serum cholesterol and markedly raised serum triglycerides
    B He is most likely to have type IIa hyperlipidaemia
    C Nephrotic syndrome is a recognised cause of this condition
    D The serum is likely to be milky
    E This patient is at risk of pancreatitis

6.21 A 12-year-old boy was referred because a random screening test had shown hypercalcaemia. He felt well in himself. He had no previous medical history and was not on any medication. His father had a similar problem and had been operated on some years ago. There were no abnormalities to be found on examination.

Bloods   Calcium   2.92   Phosphate 0.8

              ALP   500   Albumin   40

              PTH   1.3

Calcium/creatinine excretion <0.01

The most appropriate treatment for this patient is:

    A calcitonin
    B no treatment
    C parathyroidectomy
    D prednisolone
    F sodium pamidronate

6.22 Dipstick testing of urine for the presence of glucose had been used as a screening test for diabetes mellitus; 800 patients were tested for glucosuria, of whom 200 who tested positive were later diagnosed as having diabetes mellitus and there were 50 false-positives. The positive predictive value of this test is:

A 200/250
B 200/325
C 425/550
D 425/475
E 625/800

6.23 A 45-year-old man presented with impotence and breasts that had become enlarged. This had been going on over the past 3 months but he was too embarrassed to tell anyone. He drank 3 units of alcohol per day and smoked 20 cigarettes a day but was not on any medication. His only other symptom was longstanding painful knees.

On examination he had palmar erythema and gynaecomastia. There was some ankle oedema but no lymphadenopathy. Pulse was 72 regular and blood pressure 140/85. Chest and cardiovascular examination were normal. He had 3 cm hepatomegaly. Genital examination revealed small testes. Knee examination was normal.

Bloods	Hb	13.9	WCC	4.7
	Platelets	249	Na	142
	K	4.6	Urea	5.4
	Creatinine	97	Bilirubin	20
	Albumin	35	Protein	67
	ALT	45	ALP	100
	GGT	110	Calcium	2.20
	Phosphate	0.9	Glucose	12.1

Urinalysis Glucose 1+, no protein

The most likely diagnosis is:

A alcoholic liver disease
B diabetic neuropathy
C idiopathic haemochromatosis
D osteomalacia
E primary sclerosing cholangitis

6.24 A 16-year-old boy presented with 3-day history of bleeding gums and generalised purpura. On examination he had a temperature of 39.1°C. He had bilateral cervical lymphadenopathy and palpable splenomegaly.

Bloods	Hb	13.1	WCC	2.9
	Platelets	30		

Blood film Atypical lymphocytes

The most helpful test to confirm the diagnosis would be:

    A bone marrow aspirate and trephine
    B cytogenetics
    C gum biopsy
    D lymph node biopsy
    E monospot test

6.25 A 19-year-old man was referred because of progressive weakness in the lower limbs. His problems started a year ago when he found that he was walking like a 'drunkard' and noticed 'clawing' of his feet. Slurring of speech and tremor followed this. He was adopted and knew nothing about his family.

    On examination he had a mild kyphosis and pes cavus. On shaking hands he was noted to have an intention tremor. He was fully orientated and mental test score was 10/10. He had difficulty pronouncing poly-syllabic words. Cranial nerve examination revealed no abnormalities and his pupils were normal. Apart from his intention tremor his upper limbs were normal. There was weakness of both lower limbs, with increased tone and reduced power; knee and ankle reflexes were absent but plantar responses were extensor. Pinprick sensation was intact but vibration sense and proprioception were reduced. He was unable to perform heel-shin movements and Romberg's sign was positive. The most likely diagnosis is:

    A Charcot–Marie–Tooth disease
    B Friedreich's ataxia
    C multiple sclerosis
    D subacute combined degeneration of the cord
    E tabes dorsalis

6.26 A 33-year-old farm worker was referred because of fatigue, progressive shortness of breath and productive cough for over the past 6 months His breathing was worse during the day but improved before going to sleep. He had normal appetite but had lost 3 kilograms over this time. His exercise tolerance was reduced to 200 metres. There was no chest pain or palpitations. He had no previous medical history and was not on any medication. He did not smoke or drink alcohol.

    On examination there was no clubbing, cyanosis, oedema or lymph-adenopathy. His temperature was 37.3°C, pulse 100 regular and blood pressure 130/85. His JVP was not elevated and both heart sounds were normal. There were bilateral inspiratory crackles but there was no wheeze. Abdominal examination was normal.

Bloods	Hb	13.1	WCC	9.7
	Neutrophils	6.8	Lymphocytes	2.0
	Eosinophils	0.3	Platelets	239
	Na	140	K	4.7
	Urea	5.9	Creatinine	98
	Protein	65	Albumin	35
	Bilirubin	10	ALT	20
	ALP	78	Calcium	2.22

ANCA Negative

Lung function tests	Absolute	Predicted (%)
FEV_1	2.3	56
FVC	2.5	54
TLC	3.6	62
DLCO	12.3	56
KCO	3.3	48

Chest X-ray Bilateral patchy infiltrates

The most likely diagnosis is:

   A allergic bronchopulmonary alveolitis
   B bronchial asthma
   C Churg–Strauss syndrome
   D extrinsic allergic alveolitis
   E Goodpasture's syndrome

6.27 A 61-year-old man known to suffer with Raynaud's phenomenon and rheumatoid arthritis was referred with rash on both legs, present for the past 2 months. He also complained of decreased sensation and pain in both his legs but no problems walking. Over the past week he had passed blood in his urine. His appetite had decreased and he had lost weight. 10 years ago he contracted hepatitis C through a blood transfusion abroad. He was on no medication.

On examination he was apyrexial. His pulse was 88 regular and blood pressure 154/87. His JVP was not elevated and heart sounds were normal. His chest was clear. Abdominal examination revealed hepatomegaly. He had normal lower limb tone and power but absent ankle and plantar reflexes. There was decreased sensation to light touch and pinprick up to the level of mid-shin. The knee and ankle joints were tender but not inflamed. The rash on the legs was purpuric.

Bloods	Hb	11.9	MCV	92.4
	WCC	7.6	Platelets	459
	Na	138	K	4.8
	Urea	13.8	Creatinine	160
	Protein	74	Albumin	38
	Bilirubin	25	ALT	65
	ALP	100	ESR	65
	CRP	58	C3	80
	C4	8		

Rheumatoid factor	1 in 640
Antinuclear antibody	Negative
ANCA	Negative
Hepatitis A, B serology	Negative
Hepatitis C serology	Positive
Urine dipstick	Blood 2+, protein 3+
Chest X-ray	Normal

The most likely diagnosis is:

    A microscopic polyangitis
    B mixed cryoglobulinaemia
    C polyarteritis nodosa
    D systemic lupus erythematosus
    E Wegener's granulomatosis

6.28 This 16-year-old girl was admitted with a 1-day history of headache, neck stiffness and photophobia. She had a temperature of 38.5°C, pulse 110 regular and blood pressure 96/50. A lumbar puncture was undertaken and Gram stain analysis was performed on the CSF (Figure 6.28). See plate section.

The most likely organism to have caused this is:

    A *Escherichia coli*
    B *Haemophilus influenzae*
    C *Mycobacterium tuberculosis*
    D *Neisseria meningitidis*
    E *Streptococcus pneumoniae*

6.29 An 83-year-old man complained of pain in his legs for 4 months (Figure 6.29). See plate section.

The X-ray findings are most consistent with:

A congenital syphilis
B hyperparathyroidism
C osteomalacia
D Paget's disease of bone
E sarcoidosis

6.30 A 57-year-old woman was referred because of severe pain in her hands (Figure 6.30). See plate section.

The X-ray findings would be most consistent with:

A gout
B hyperparathyroidism
C psoriatic arthropathy
D rheumatoid arthritis
E systemic sclerosis

6.31 A 14-year-old Nigerian girl was referred feeling lethargic and with pain and swelling in both knees for the past week. She had returned from visiting her family in Nigeria 2 weeks ago. While on holiday she had developed a sore throat. She had no previous medical history and was on no medication.

On examination she had a temperature of 37.4°C. Her pulse was 66 regular and blood pressure 90/64. Her JVP was not elevated and she had an additional heard sound but no murmurs. Her chest was clear. Abdominal examination was normal. Both knees were hot, tender and swollen but there was no focal neurological abnormality.

Bloods	Hb	12.4	WCC	13.5
	Neutrophils	11.0	Platelets	330
	Na	136	K	4.5
	Urea	2.5	Creatinine	58
	Albumin	38	Protein	75
	Bilirubin	12	ALP	380
	ALT	24	Calcium	2.40
	Phosphate	0.98	ESR	120
	CRP	59	Urate	0.16
Rheumatoid factor		Negative		
Antinuclear antibody		Negative		

Hb electrophoresis	Normal	
Antistreptolysin O titre	1/160	
Hepatitis A, B, C serology	Negative	
Synovial fluid	WCC 350	50% polymorphs
	No growth	
ECG	1st degree AV block	
Chest X-ray	Normal	

The most likely diagnosis is:

    A infective endocarditis
    B Kawasaki disease
    C rheumatic fever
    D Still's disease
    E systemic lupus erythematosus

6.32 A 67-year-old man admitted with an inferior MI 2 days ago developed palpitations and shortness of breath. As the doctor approached the patient he became pale, cold and clammy. The cardiac monitor showed the following trace:

Assuming he improved after defibrillation, the next step in the immediate management of this patient would be:

A amiodarone infusion
B intravenous atropine
C lignocaine infusion
D magnesium infusion
E temporary pacing wire

6.33 A 70-year-old man was referred because of a 2-month history of a pruritic rash affecting the axillae, upper abdomen and neck. He had no previous medical problems and was not on any medication (Figure 6.33). See plate section.

The most likely diagnosis is:

A bullous pemphigoid
B dermatitis herpetiformis
C epidermolysis bullosa
D pemphigus vulgaris
E scalded skin syndrome

6.34 A 45-year-old businessman was referred with progressive weight gain and lethargy. He smoked 20 cigarettes a day and drank 3 units of alcohol in the evening. He had a normal appetite. He found his job very stressful and was having some marital difficulties.

On examination he was plethoric and obese. There was some ankle oedema and bruising of his skin. His pulse was 98 regular and his blood pressure was 165/90. His chest was clear. Abdominal examination was normal.

	Urinary free cortisol (nmol/24 h)	Cortisol/nmol/l) 9 am	midnight	ACTH/ng/l) 9 am
Basal	400	900	150	50
0.5 mg qds dexamethasone suppression test (48 h)		720		
2 mg qds dexamethasone suppression test (48 h)		345		

The most likely diagnosis in this patient is:

A ACTH-secreting adrenal adenoma
B cortisol-secreting adrenal adenoma
C ectopic ACTH secretion
D pituitary-dependent adenoma
E pseudo-Cushing's disease due to alcohol

6.35 A 28-year-old woman was referred because she wanted to start a family. Her father suffered from haemophilia A but her mother had no clinical evidence of the disease. Her husband had also been tested and had a normal genotype. Her risk of having a son with haemophilia A is:

A 0%
B 25%
C 50%
D 75%
E 100%

6.36 A 45-year-old publican was admitted with severe right-sided abdominal pain for the past 2 days, which radiated to the back and woke him from sleep. It came and went in severe spasms with no relieving factors. There was also some haematuria. He drank 2 units of alcohol a day, although he had cut down his intake. Over the past four months he had lost weight and had a decreased appetite. His stools were foul smelling and were difficult to flush away.

On examination he had a temperature of 37.4°C, pulse 88 regular and blood pressure 130/78. He was tender over the right loin but had no guarding. There was no organomegaly and bowel sounds were present. Rectal examination revealed steatorrhoea.

Bloods	Hb	13.5	WCC	12.3
	Neutrophils	10.0	Platelets	325
	Na	139	K	4.5
	Urea	5.6	Creatinine	100
	Albumin	35	Protein	67
	Calcium	2.01	Phosphate	0.80
	Amylase	100		

Urinalysis Blood 2+

Abdominal X-ray Three small right renal calculi seen

The likely composition of the renal calculi in this patient would be:

A cystine
B oxalate
C phosphate
D urate
E xanthine

6.37 A 77-year-old man was admitted with an acute facial and left limb weakness. He had no previous medical history. He smoked 30 cigarettes per day and drank 4 units of alcohol per night.

On examination he was unable to close his right eye and the angle of his mouth on the right was drooping down. He was unable to raise his right eyebrow. Ear examination was normal. There was left-sided weakness of his upper and lower limbs. Tone was increased and power was reduced. His right plantar response was flexor and his left plantar was extensor. No sensory abnormalities could be detected. The likely cause of the facial weakness is:

A Bell's palsy
B Foster Kennedy syndrome due to cerebral tumour
C right middle cerebral artery occlusion
D right posterior inferior cerebellar artery thrombosis
E right-sided pontine infarction

6.38 A 34-year-old man was admitted with severe shortness of breath and cough productive of yellow sputum. This was his third admission this year with chest problems. He was a heavy smoker. He took nebulised salbutamol and ipratropium bromide but did not have home oxygen therapy and had not required ventilation in the past. He had never been exposed to asbestos.

On examination he was breathless at rest. His temperature was 37.4°C, pulse 98 regular and blood pressure 135/86. His respiratory rate was 28 breaths/min and he had bilateral wheeze on chest auscultation. There was also 2 cm non-tender hepatomegaly. The admitting doctor considered a possible diagnosis of α_1-antitrypsin deficiency.

Bloods				
Hb	14.7	WCC	12.7
Platelets	190	Na	145
K	4.3	Urea	7.5
Creatinine	110	Protein	58
Albumin	38	Bilirubin	30
ALT	34	ALP	76

Chest X-ray   Hyperinflated lung fields
Bulla in right base

Arterial blood	pH	7.38	PCO$_2$	6.7
gases on air	PO$_2$	7.8	Bicarbonate	35.2
	Base excess	8.7		

Which **ONE** of the following statements concerning this patient's condition is correct?

A Administration of influenza vaccination is contraindicated

B He is likely to develop centrilobular emphysema

C If a liver transplant for cirrhosis was performed the condition would recur in the new donor organ

D Lung function tests are likely to show a decreased FEV$_1$:FVC ratio and increased residual volume

E Patients with a phenotype of PiMM are more likely to develop emphysema

6.39 A 53-year-old man was referred with a 12-month history of abdominal pain and bloating and loose stools. He had lost 4 kg, associated with decreased appetite. His stools were semiliquid with some mucus but no blood. There was no nausea or vomiting. Recently he had also become increasingly lethargic and short of breath on exertion. He had a previous medical history of arthritis that affected various joints for a few days before resolving: hips, knees, elbows and shoulders. He only took paracetamol. He did not drink alcohol or smoke. He had no recent travel abroad.

On examination he was thin and his skin was hyperpigmented but there was no rash. There was cervical lymphadenopathy. His temperature was 37.2°C, pulse 90 regular and blood pressure 120/78. His JVP was not elevated and heart sounds were normal. There was dullness to percussion at both lung bases. His abdomen was soft and mildly tender. There was no organomegaly and rectal examination was normal. Neurological examination was normal. Left knee joint was mildly swollen and inflamed but there was no effusion clinically.

Bloods	Hb	11.9	MCV	100.2
	WCC	4.6	Platelets	340
	Na	136	K	3.9
	Urea	5.3	Creatinine	100
	Protein	64	Albumin	34
	Bilirubin	20	ALT	28
	ALP	120	Calcium	1.89
	Phosphate	0.71	ESR	35
	CRP	42	Amylase	40
Rheumatoid factor	Negative			
Chest X-ray	Bilateral pleural effusions			

Abdominal ultrasound   Normal

Upper GI endoscopy   Normal

Colonoscopy   Normal

The most likely diagnosis is:

    A amyloidosis
    B ankylosing spondylitis
    C carcinoid syndrome
    D coeliac disease
    E Whipple's disease

6.40 This 55-year-old man was referred for endoscopy because of inter-mittent dysphagia. A fixed lesion was seen at endoscopy (Figure 6.40). See plate section.

The endoscopic findings were constant and are consistent with:

    A achalasia
    B Barrett's oesophagus
    C benign oesophageal stricture
    D oesophageal carcinoma
    E Schatzki ring

6.41 A 27-year-old man known to suffer from HIV and to be a heavy drinker was brought in confused and drowsy. He could not say whether he had suffered any trauma to his head.

    On examination his temperature was 37.1°C, pulse 92 regular and blood pressure 130/88. Cardiovascular and respiratory examination were normal. His GCS score was 14/15. Pupils were equal and reactive to light. He was unable to name objects and was disorientated in time, place and person. Plantar responses were extensor on the left and absent on the right (Figure 6.41). See plate section.

The following **TWO** diagnoses that can be made from the scan are:

    A acute right cerebral infarct
    B acute right extradural haemorrhage
    C acute right intracerebral haemorrhage
    D acute right subdural haemorrhage
    E cerebral abscess
    F cerebral toxoplasmosis
    G chronic right cerebral infarct
    H chronic right subdural haemorrhage
    I midline shift
    J subarachnoid haemorrhage

6.42 A 50-year-old man known to suffer with muscle weakness and arthritis was referred with a rash on both hands. There was a rash on the face that involved the eyelids (Figure 6.42). See plate section.

The most likely diagnosis is:

    A dermatomyositis
    B porphyria cutanea tarda
    C rheumatoid arthritis
    D systemic lupus erythematosus
    E systemic sclerosis

6.43 A 25-year-old woman presented with a 3-month history of headaches, palpitations and sweating. She had been started on bendroflumethiazide (bendrofluazide) because she was found to be hypertensive but that had not helped her symptoms. She had no previous medical history. She smoked 10 cigarettes per day but did not drink alcohol.

On examination her pulse was 100 regular and blood pressure 200/130. JVP was not elevated and heart sounds were normal. Her chest was clear. She had no neck swelling. Abdominal examination was normal. Fundoscopy revealed flame-shaped haemorrhages and cotton wool spots.

Bloods	Hb	15.6	WCC	6.7
	Platelets	400	Na	140
	K	4.0	Urea	5.0
	Creatinine	98	TSH	2.5
	Free T$_4$	20	Glucose	7.5

Chest X-ray Enlarged heart

ECG Sinus tachycardia

Voltage criteria for left ventricular hypertrophy

The most likely diagnosis is

    A carcinoid syndrome
    B Conn's syndrome
    C Cushing's syndrome
    D phaeochromocytoma
    E T$_3$ thyrotoxicosis

6.44 A 20-year-old man presented with a 2-week history of abdominal pain and bloody diarrhoea. He was opening his bowels over eight times a day and his stools were 'almost liquid'. He had decreased appetite and had lost over 3 kg in weight. He had not travelled abroad recently or come into contact with anyone else who was ill. He had no previous medical history. He did not smoke or drink and was not on any medication.

On examination his temperature was 37.8°C, pulse 110 regular and blood pressure 95/50. He had generalised abdominal tenderness. Rectal examination revealed fresh blood.

Bloods

Hb	10.5	WCC	12.5
Neutrophils	10.2	Platelets	500
Na	140	K	3.9
Urea	5.9	Creatinine	100
Albumin	28	Protein	56
ALT	25	ALP	70
Amylase	49	ESR	45
CRP	200		

Chest X-ray Normal

Abdominal X-ray Some large bowel dilatation; no obstruction

Which **ONE** of the following statements regarding management is true?

A Await the results of urgent colonoscopy before starting treatment
B Consider colectomy if there is no overnight improvement
C Start intravenous hydrocortisone
D Transfuse at least 2 units of blood
E Treat with intravenous antibiotics after stool cultures have been taken

6.45 A 48-year-old man was referred with sleep problems. He complained of excessive sleepiness and falling asleep at the wheel of his car. At night he had woken up and felt his whole body paralysed. On a number of occasions he had collapsed without warning but with no loss of consciousness and these attacks lasted a few minutes. There was no previous medical history. He did not smoke or drink alcohol. He had not been on any long-haul flights recently.

On examination he looked well. There were no clinical abnormalities to find on examination and his body mass index was 25. The most likely diagnosis is:

A bruxism
B complex partial epilepsy
C idiopathic insomnia
D narcolepsy
E obstructive sleep apnoea

6.46 A 64-year-old woman complained of headaches. She also had pain in her back and hips (Figure 6.46) See plate section.

The most likely diagnosis is:

    A hypoparathyroidism
    B multiple myeloma
    C osteoporosis
    D Paget's disease of bone
    E Sturge–Weber syndrome

6.47 A 12-year-old boy was referred to the dermatology clinic (Figure 6.47). See plate section.

The dermatological sign elicited here is:

    A cutis hyperelastica
    B cutis laxa
    C dermatographia
    D Nikolsky's sign
    E pathergy

6.48 A 30-year-old woman developed a non-tender swelling in her neck, followed by tiredness, palpitations and sweating. She was 6-weeks postpartum. She had no previous medical history and had had no recent illnesses. She was not on any medication.

    On examination she had bilateral lid lag. Her skin was moist and she had palmar erythema. Her pulse was 110 regular and blood pressure 145/90. She had a smooth non-tender goitre.

Bloods	Hb	13.5	WCC	9.5
	Platelets	230	ESR	9
	TSH	0.01	Free T$_4$	35

24-hour radioactive ^{131}I uptake scan   <1% uptake after 24 hours

The most likely diagnosis is:

    A De Quervain's thyroiditis
    B Graves' disease
    C postpartum thyroiditis
    D sick euthyroid syndrome
    E solitary toxic adenoma

6.49 A 45-year-old man with cirrhosis presented with ascites. This was his fourth presentation and it had been drained each time because of resistance to diuretics.

    On examination he looked cachexic but apart from ascites there were no other abnormalities to be found. He was not encephalopathic and had never had spontaneous bacterial peritonitis. He was assessed for liver transplantation.

Which **ONE** of the following would **NOT** be a contraindication for liver transplantation?

    A Alcoholic liver disease and drinking until hospital admission.
    B Dukes' A colonic carcinoma
    C HIV infection
    D Portal vein and superior mesenteric vein thrombosis
    E Primary sclerosing cholangitis that has now developed cholangiocarcinoma

6.50 A 13-year-old boy was referred because of headaches and fits which had been occurring on and off for a number of years (Figure 6.50). See plate section

The X-ray findings would be consistent with:

    A hypoparathyroidism
    B Laurence–Moon–Biedl syndrome
    C neurofibromatosis
    D Sturge–Weber syndrome
    E tuberous sclerosis

6.51 A 14-year-old boy presented with 'collapse'. He did not lose consciousness and did not convulse. Prior to this he had been getting tingling in hands for a number of years but had never received any treatment. He had no other medical problems and was not on any medication.

    On examination he looked unwell. There appeared to be some darkening of the buccal mucosa in his mouth. His pulse was 100 regular and blood pressure 95/60. There were no other abnormalities on clinical examination.

Bloods	Hb	12.5	WCC	8.3
	Platelets	345	Na	130
	K	6.2	Urea	4.3
	Creatinine	50	Glucose	2.8
	Calcium	1.95	Albumin	40
	PTH	0.4		

The most likely diagnosis is:

    A MEN 1 syndrome
    B MEN 2A syndrome
    C MEN 2B syndrome
    D APS 1
    E APS 2

6.52 A 30-year-old woman was referred with a 6-month history of chronic diarrhoea. She had a normal appetite and no weight loss. There was no previous medical history or significant family history and she was on no medication. A diagnosis of irritable bowel syndrome was suspected.

Which **ONE** of the following symptoms would **NOT** be typical of this condition?

   A Feeling of incomplete evacuation
   B Passing loose, watery stools
   C Passing mucus in the stools
   D Severe bloating
   E Waking from sleep to open bowels

6.53 A 20-year-old man presented with a sore throat to his general practitioner who diagnosed tonsillitis and treated him with amoxicillin. Three days later he re-presented to his general practitioner complaining of haematuria. He reported no joint pain or rash. He had no other medical problems and was on no other medication.

   On examination he was apyrexial, with some cervical lymphadenopathy and red inflamed tonsils. The rest of the physical examination was normal.

Bloods	Hb	13.0	WCC	8.5
	Platelets	270	Na	138
	K	4.5	Urea	2.8
	Creatinine	68	Protein	70
	Albumin	40	CRP	25

Urinanalysis Protein 1+, red cells 1+, blood 1+, no white cells

Red cell casts and dysmorphic red cells

Chest X-ray Normal

The most likely diagnosis is:

   A acute interstitial nephritis secondary to amoxicillin treatment
   B Henoch–Schönlein purpura
   C IgA nephropathy
   D infectious mononucleosis
   E poststreptococcal glomerulonephritis

6.54 A 45-year-old man presented to Accident & Emergency with pyrexia, malaise and abdominal pain. He returned from Nigeria 10 days ago (Figure 6.54). See plate section.

The organism seen in the film is:

A *Plasmodium falciparum*
B *Loa loa*
C *Leishmania donovani*
D *Trypanosoma brucei gambiense*
E *Schistosoma haematobium*

6.55 A 49-year-old man with advanced disease had a biopsy to assess prognosis (Figure 6.55). See plate section.

Which **ONE** of the following prognostic scoring systems could be applied to this patient?

A Ann Arbor
B Rockall
C Childs–Pugh
D Dukes'
E Breslow

6.56 A 62-year-old man was referred feeling unwell. He had just finished a course of chemotherapy for lymphoma. He had no cough or urinary symptoms but reported malaise and decreased appetite for the past 2 days.

On examination his temperature was 38.5°C, pulse 100 regular and blood pressure 100/78. His chest was clear and abdominal examination was normal. There was no focal neurological defect and plantar responses were flexor. Examination of the oropharynx was also normal.

Bloods	Hb	12.1	WCC	1.4
	Neutrophils	0.9	Lymphocytes	0.5
	Platelets	130	INR	1.1
	Na	139	K	4.8
	Urea	10.6	Creatinine	139
	Protein	78	Albumin	31
	Bilirubin	12	ALT	22
	ALP	120	CRP	40

Chest X-ray Normal

Urinananlysis No WCC, no protein

The most appropriate treatment for this patient is:

A ceftazidime and fluconazole
B cefuroxime and metronidazole
C rifampicin, isoniazid and pyrazinamide
D trazocin and gentamicin
E vancomycin and fusidic acid

6.57 A 63-year-old woman was referred because she had cervical lymph-adenopathy and a palpable spleen. For blood film see plate 6.57.

The most likely diagnosis is:

- A acute lymphoblastic leukaemia
- B acute myeloid leukaemia
- C chronic lymphocytic leukaemia
- D chronic myeloid leukaemia
- E infectious mononucleosis

6.58 A 54-year-old man was being assessed for a coronary artery bypass graft. He had a previous history of intermittent claudication and hyper-tension but was on no medication. He was a heavy smoker. He was noted to have cholesterol 8.2, urea 15 and creatinine 210.

On examination his pulse was 90 regular and blood pressure 170/100. His JVP was not elevated and chest and heart sounds were normal. Abdominal examination was normal but there were bilateral femoral bruits. Fundoscopy revealed flame-shaped haemorrhages and silver-wiring.

Urinanalysis Normal

Renal ultrasound Left kidney 9 cm, right kidney 10.9 cm

No hydronephrosis or extrarenal masses

The next most helpful test to aid diagnosis of the renal findings would be:

- A DMSA scan
- B Doppler ultrasound
- C MAG 3 scan
- D magnetic resonance angiography
- E renal biopsy

6.59 A 43-year-old HIV-positive man was referred because of chronic watery diarrhoea that had been going on for 5 months. He also had associated abdominal pain, decreased appetite and weight loss of 6 kg in that time period. He had no other medical problems and was on no medication.

He appeared cachexic but the rest of his physical examination was unremarkable.

Bloods	Hb	12.8	WCC	4.2
	Platelets	190		
CD4	300			
Viral load	12,000			

Of the following the most likely cause of his symptoms is:

A Cryptosporidia
B Cytomegalovirus colitis
C Microsporidia
D Mycobacterium avium intracellulare
E Non-Hodgkin's lymphoma

6.60 A 34-year-old Algerian refugee was referred because of malaise, ankle swelling and heavy proteinuria for the past month. In the past he had suffered from recurrent elbow and knee joint pain and intermittent abdominal pain. He had no surviving family members. He smoked 15 cigarettes per day but did not drink alcohol. He was on no medication.

On examination he had bilateral pitting oedema up to the thighs. He was apyrexial, pulse 79 regular and blood pressure 125/84. His JVP was not elevated and heart sounds were normal. There was dullness at both lung bases. Abdominal and musculoskeletal examination was normal.

Bloods	Hb	10.6	MCV	93.4
	WCC	7.9	Platelets	346
	Na	140	K	4.8
	Urea	8.2	Creatinine	128
	Protein	50	Albumin	22
	ESR	40	CRP	26
	C_3	80	C_4	30

Urinanalysis Protein 4+, no blood, no red cells, no white cells

24-hour urinary protein collection 12.7 g/L

The most helpful test to determine the diagnosis is:

A antinuclear antibody
B protein electrophoresis
C rectal biopsy
D renal biopsy
E serum cryoglobulins

Answers

6.1 **C**** Patients with inferior or inferoposterior MI are at risk of infarcting the right ventricle. The clinical presentation is of a patient who becomes acutely unwell, hypotensive, with an elevated JVP and clear lung fields. An ECG will usually show ST elevation in the inferior leads (II, III and aVF) and ST elevation in V4R–V6R. The correct management of these patients is to fluid resuscitate with possible inotropic support to ensure high filling pressures. Rupture of the interventricular septum to produce acute ventricular septal defect, and rupture of the papillary muscles to produce acute mitral regurgitation may also cause hypotension and elevated JVP. However, one would expect to hear a murmur and the development of acute pulmonary oedema. Cardiac tamponade is very difficult to diagnose but should be suspected if heart sounds are difficult to hear, there is an elevated JVP, pulsus paradoxus and a globular heart on chest X-ray.

6.2 **E**** The ECG shows ST elevation in leads II, III and aVF with ST depression in V_{1-3} consistent with an inferoposterior MI.

6.3 **B*** This young girl may well have taken amphetamines or 'Ecstasy' or MDMA (methylenedioxymetamphetamine) while in the nightclub, which could account for her malignant hyperpyrexia, acute renal failure, imminent disseminated intravascular coagulopathy and decreased conscious level. If her creatinine kinase were measured it would be very raised consistent with rhabdomyolysis in which myoglobin is released; hence, urine dipstick and microscopy will reveal blood but no red cells. The mainstay of treatment is rehydration and alkalinisation of urine. Furosemide (frusemide) acidifies urine and may enhance myoglobin tubular damage. With rhabdomyolysis there is a risk of compartment syndrome and so fasciotomy may be necessary.

6.4 **C**** This patient has acanthosis nigricans, which is a rare, darkly pigmented, velvety thickening of flexural skin. It can be associated with insulin resistance, obesity and various endocrinopathies such insulin dependent diabetes, Cushing's syndrome, polycystic ovary disease and thyroid disease. In the absence of these, malignant disease should be excluded. Intra-abdominal adenocarcinoma should be suspected: stomach, colon, pancreas, gallbladder and oesophagus. Renal cell carcinoma is not an association.

6.5 **A*** During pregnancy women may develop a goitre. There is an increase of total thyroxine but normal levels of free T_4 and free T_3. Virus-induced subacute thyroiditis may cause transient thyrotoxicosis but is usually associated with thyroid tenderness and, unlike other forms of hyperthyroidism, reduced radioactive iodine uptake.

6.6 **B**** ARR is the absolute amount by which β-interferon reduces the risk of relapse at the end of 5 years. As patients are randomly assigned, there are 1000 patients in each group.

RR of relapse in β-interferon group = 20/1000 = 0.02

RR of relapse in placebo group = 100/1000 = 0.1

ARR = 0.1–0.02 = 0.08

6.7 **D*** This patient has decompensated liver disease, most probably due to alcoholic liver disease. Clinically he is in renal failure, although biochemically it might not appear that way. If left to continue he will almost certainly develop hepatorenal syndrome. Hepatorenal syndrome is a form of acute tubular necrosis where the kidneys have failed due to hepatic failure. Should the liver be transplanted, the kidneys will work normally. This patient is oliguric and so restricting fluid will only make his renal failure worse. These patients have enough sodium in their body but an excess of water, giving a dilutional hyponatremia. The water logging effect is due to a combination of hypoalbuminaemia, arteriovenous shunting, and splanchnic vasodilatation; fluid is lost into the extravascular space, triggering the renin–angiotensin–aldosterone system to secrete more aldosterone, in turn producing more sodium retention. To give saline would only add to this vicious cycle. If patients are becoming oliguric then a CVP line should be inserted and colloid should be given as maintenance fluid. If that should fail, pressor agents like terlipressin should be considered. Lactulose will help clear the bowel and so prevent constipation and alter the bowel pH. Blood transfusions should be avoided unless necessary as they can trigger encephalopathy. Regular diazepam should not be given in a patient with hypoxia but may be given cautiously if fits or delirium tremens develop.

6.8 **C**** G6PD is an essential enzyme that prevents denaturation of haemoglobin and the cell membrane under periods of oxidative stress. Deficiency results in the production of Heinz bodies and reticulocytosis. Type A G6PD deficiency disease is associated with acute haemolysis after the ingestion of certain drugs like antimalarials, sulphonamides and phenacetin. Type B G6PD deficiency disease tends to affect individuals of Mediterranean origin and results in severe intravascular haemolysis with exposure to fava beans. Pyruvate kinase deficiency is associated with extravascular haemolysis, splenomegaly and prickle cells on blood film. The Coombs' test detects autoimmune haemolytic anaemia.

6.9 **D**** This slide is stained with Ziehl–Nielsen stain and shows clumped red-purple bacilli on a green background. This is characteristic of *Mycobacterium* TB. *Pneumocystis carinii* would stain with silver stain.

6.10 **D**** Pregnant mothers with HIV should be given anti-HIV treatment during pregnancy even if they are asymptomatic; the choice of drugs will depend on the viral load, as the higher this is the more drugs will be given. Risk of vertical transmission is greatest at the intrapartum period and so elective Caesarean section should be planned. Breast-feeding can transmit the virus and should be avoided. The baby should be given AZT for the first 4–6 weeks of life to reduce the risk of vertical transmission.

6.11 **A***** The diagnosis is Guillain–Barré syndrome or postinfective poly-neuropathy with progressive ascending peripheral neuropathy following a viral infection. The CSF protein is very high and this would not be found with the other conditions.

6.12 **D, H*** This patient is diabetic and has a ring of hard exudates close to the macula. There is also a boat-shaped lesion characteristic of preretinal haemorrhage/subhyaloid haemorrhage, which is due to bleeding into the small space between the retina and posterior vitreous.

6.13 **D*** The most obvious abnormalities on his blood picture are pancytopenia and hypokalaemia. The patient is on chemotherapy, which could include platinum compounds like cisplatin. Side effects of cisplatin include hypo-magnesaemia, myelosuppression, gastrointestinal disturbances, nephro-toxicity and ototoxicity. Ectopic ACTH secretion occurs with small cell bronchial carcinomas (not squamous cell) and gives rise to hypokalaemic alkalosis.

6.14 **C**** This patient is likely to have Sjögren's syndrome, as suggested by dry mouth, Raynaud's phenomenon, the presence of other autoimmune disease and confirmatory blood tests. The positive serological tests associated with Sjögren's syndrome are rheumatoid factor (80–95%), positive antinuclear antibodies (90%), and raised anti-Ro and anti-La antibodies (50–90%). Classically patients also present with dry eyes and bilateral parotid gland swelling. The autoimmune profile is not consistent with systemic sclerosis and polymyositis. Mixed connective tissue disease is an overlap syndrome of rheumatoid arthritis, systemic lupus erythematosus, scleroderma and myosi-tis; such patients lack other autoantibodies like anti-Ro, anti-La and anti-DS DNA.

6.15 **D**** This picture shows Hutchinson's teeth, which appear as barrel-shaped upper incisors. Normal incisors narrow towards the base, Hutchinson's incisors are broad at the base and narrow towards the cutting surface. 'Hutchinson's triad' consists of Hutchinson's teeth, inner ear deafness and interstitial keratitis, which could account for the temporary loss of vision. This triad and saddle-shaped nose are reliable signs of congenital syphilis.

6.16 **D**** There are bilateral confluent shadows. Caplan's syndrome is coal worker's pneumoconiosis associated with rheumatoid arthritis; there is no mention of the latter. There is no pleural thickening to suggest meso-thelioma. The apparent absence of a goitre does not exclude a thyroid carcinoma that has metastasised to the lung. Teratoma and renal cell carcinoma metastases could also give this X-ray picture.

6.17 B** The X-ray shows gas gangrene in the young boy's thigh. The most likely organism is *C. septicum. C. perfringens* can also cause gas gangrene.

6.18 A** This patient has HOCM. This is a primary heart muscle disorder characterised by inappropriate myocardial hypertrophy of a non-dilated left ventricle and often associated with a degree of outflow tract obstruction. Syncope is usually exertional and is due to a combination of ischaemia, arrhythmias, outflow tract obstruction and poor diastolic ventricular filling. Drugs such as diuretics, nitrates and ACE inhibitors reduce preload and decrease chamber size, making the condition worse. They may increase the outflow tract gradient and, along with inotropic agents like digoxin, can induce arrhythmias that can worsen diastolic function. β-Blockers and verapamil slow the heart rate, increase the diastolic filling period and reduce outflow obstruction.

6.19 B** This patient's ECG shows atrial flutter with 4:1 block. It is unusual to develop idiopathic atrial flutter, but it may be caused by any of the causes of atrial fibrillation. Drugs like sotalol, flecainide, propafenone and disopyramide are effective in terminating flutter; adenosine can often slow the heart rate down to reveal flutter as the underlying rhythm but does not usually termi-nate it. This patient is not haemodynamically compromised so DC cardio-version is not indicated. As there is the risk of thromboembolic event like stroke, he should be anticoagulated especially if cardioversion is going to be attempted. A pacemaker is not indicated.

6.20 B* This patient has eruptive xanthoma. These are small papules or nodules, which have a predilection for the gluteal regions and extensor surfaces. They are indicative of hypertriglyceridaemia and such patients are likely to have raised chylomycrons and very low density lipoproteins. The serum cholesterol may be normal or slightly elevated. Acute pancreatitis is a very serious risk. Eruptive xanthomas are associated with types I, IV and V hyper-lipidaemia where triglycerides are raised. Nephrotic syndrome, diabetes, gout and hypothyroidism are all associated with hypertriglyceridaemia. Type IIa hyperlipidaemia is associated with raised cholesterol only.

6.21 B* This patient has familial autosomal dominant hypercalcaemic hypo-calciuria. It is a rare but benign condition that can be confused with primary hyperparathyroidism, leading to inappropriate surgery, as may have happened to his father. Patients have a normal parathyroid hormone level and calcium/creatinine excretion <0.01. The seemingly high ALP is normal for a boy of his age.

6.22 A** The positive predictive value is the probability that a patient who tests positive really does have the condition.

	Diabetes +	Diabetes −	
Glucosuria +	200 (a)	50 (b)	250

Positive predictive value = a/a+b = 200/250 = 0.80

6.23 C* Signs of chronic liver disease, arthralgia and an elevated glucose are suggestive of haemochromatosis, which can be primary/idiopathic, or secondary to iron overload conditions like alcoholic liver disease. Both conditions may present in a number of ways: bronze diabetes (partly due to iron deposition in the liver and increased insulin resistance), congestive cardiac failure (due to cardiomyopathy), hypogonadism, and arthropathy (due to pseudogout, which primarily affects the metacarpals, wrists, hips and knees). He does not have a history suggestive of alcoholic liver disease. He is diabetic, but even if he were to have neuropathy this would not explain arthralgia, gynaecomastia and palmar erythema.

6.24 E** Infectious mononucleosis is a viral illness due to Epstein–Barr virus. If infectious mononucleosis were suspected, as suggested by the atypical lymphocytes, then the monospot test would be the confirmatory test. A lymph node biopsy would be a useful test if the monospot test was negative and lymphoma was suspected. Cytogenetics and bone marrow investigation would be necessary tests in the investigation of leukaemia.

6.25 B** Friedreich's ataxia is an autosomal recessive (or very rarely X-linked recessive) disorder affecting the cerebellum, spinal cord and peripheral nerves. There is pyramidal weakness in the legs. Ankle and knee reflexes may be lost owing to peripheral neuropathy. The sensory deficits are due to involvement of the dorsal columns and maybe the lateral spinothalamic tract. Other features include cardiomyopathy, optic atrophy, diabetes and dementia. Multiple sclerosis can also produce cerebellar, pyramidal and dorsal column signs but is not associated with pes cavus and absent reflexes. Tabes dorsalis can produce absent reflexes and positive Romberg's sign but only taboparesis is associated with extensor plantars. Tabes dorsalis would also be associated with Argyll Robertson pupils: small, irregular and respond to accommodation but not light.

6.26 D** Extrinsic allergic alveolitis is a type of hypersensitivity syndrome that results in a diffuse interstitial granulomatous lung disease caused by an allergic response to inhaled organic dust or chemicals; here, fungal spores are probably causing farmer's lung. This patient has progressive dyspnoea with cough, which is worse during the day, presumably when he is at work and exposed to the allergen. When he is removed from the allergen his symptoms improve. With chronic exposure, irreversible lung damage may occur. His lung function tests show a restrictive pattern (FEV$_1$:FVC ratio

92%), normal eosinophil count and lack of wheeze, which excludes asthma and allergic bronchopulmonary aspergillosis. Churg–Strauss syndrome is unlikely in a patient with a negative ANCA and lack of renal involvement. With Goodpasture's syndrome there would be a history of pulmonary haemorrhage.

6.27 B** Peripheral neuropathy, vasculitic rash, arthritis, haematuria and renal impairment suggestive of a glomerulonephritis, history of hepatitis C infection, a raised globulin, low C4 and positive rheumatoid factor are all features consistent with mixed cryoglobulinaemia. There are a number of causes of cryoglobulinaemia, including other autoimmune conditions like SLE and Wegener's granulomotosis but negative ANA and ANCA fail to support these diagnoses. Fifty per cent of patients with cryoglobulinaemia have antibodies to hepatitis C. Renal complications are common and are associated with a poorer prognosis.

6.28 E** This Gram stain shows purple Gram-positive diplococci. Gram-negative organisms would stain red. All the other organisms are Gram-negative (except TB).

6.29 D*** This is a 'sabre tibia', where the tibia is grossly bowed with sparing of the fibula; there is a pathological fracture. Although characteristic of Paget's disease, the term was originally applied to the osteitis of congenital syphilis; however, this is hardly likely to present at this age!

6.30 E** The X-ray shows terminal phalangeal resorption and soft tissue calcification. With gout, there is no calcification of tophi. Psoriatic arthropathy has a 'pencil-in-cup' deformity. There are no features of rheumatoid arthritis such as ulnar deviation. Compare this X-ray with that of hyperparathyroidism (see **4.30**).

6.31 C** This young girl presents with low-grade pyrexia, arthritis, 1st degree heart block, a possible pericardial rub, a raised ESR and antistreptolysin O titre, and a history of a sore throat. There is no single pathognomonic test for rheumatic fever but she has enough of the Jones criteria to meet this diagnosis. To diagnose rheumatic fever there needs to be evidence of streptococcal infection (history of sore throat and raised antistreptolysin O titre) and two major criteria (carditis, polyarthritis, chorea, erythema marginatum and subcutaneous nodules); or one major criterion and two minor criteria (arthralgia, fever, raised ESR or CRP, and prolonged PR interval). Still's disease is a form of juvenile rheumatoid arthritis, which would have high spiking fevers, splenomegaly, lymphadenopathy and serositis. Kawasaki disease/syndrome is a severe childhood illness that causes inflammation of blood vessels, especially coronary vessels, associated with fever, swollen hands and feet, swollen lips and tongue and lymphadenopathy. It rarely affects children aged over 8 years.

6.32 E* The cardiac monitor shows ventricular standstill followed by ventricular tachycardia. Assuming defibrillation works, he will need a temporary pacing wire as his problem is most likely to be due to bradycardia leading to ventricular fibrillation as an escape rhythm.

6.33 A** This man has symmetrical tense blisters affecting the upper part of his body, which are characteristic of bullous pemphigoid. There are linear deposits of IgG and C3 complement within the basement membrane. The condition is lethal in up to 50% of cases if left untreated but does respond to steroids. Dermatitis herpetiformis is a bullous disease associated with coeliac disease that tends to affect shoulder girdle, gluteal region, and scalp and extensor surfaces of the limbs. While it can cause burning pain and pruritus, it is not life-threatening. Pemphigus is discussed in another question (see **1.47**).

6.34 D** This patient has a form of Cushing's syndrome, as shown by the raised 24-hour urinary free cortisol and failure of the serum cortisol to normalise with a low dose dexamethasone suppression test (0.5 mg q.d.s.). The next step is to determine whether his condition is ACTH-dependent or ACTH-independent. The serum cortisol is partly suppressed when the patient is given high dose dexamethasone (2 mg q.d.s.) and is consistent with pituitary dependent adenoma.

6.35 C** Haemophilia A is an X-linked recessive disease. The patient's father must have been carrying the haemophilia gene to develop the disease. With X-linked recessive disorders all the daughters (including the patient in this case) will be obligate carriers and all the sons will be clear of the disease. If the patient has a child with an unaffected person then, as she is heterozygous for the gene, half of her sons will be unaffected and half will develop haemophilia A. Antenatal diagnosis can be undertaken in a female fetus who has a high chance of being a carrier, as well as in the male fetus, by chorionic villus sampling.

6.36 B** This patient has chronic pancreatitis. Patients with steatorrhoea have high concentrations of long chain fatty acids in their colon. These can bind to calcium salts so that there is less calcium available to bind dietary oxalate. The possible consequence of this is that more unbound oxalate can be absorbed and so lead to formation of oxalate stones.

6.37 E** He appears to have had a stroke (cerebrovascular accident) causing a left hemiplegia and, simultaneously, also causing a right lower motor neurone facial palsy with no other localising features. As it is most likely that there is a single rather than multiple lesions responsible, this localises such a lesion to the right side of the pons. There is close proximity of VII and VI but the latter has been spared. A VI nerve palsy can sometimes be a false localising sign caused by raised intracranial pressure in the Foster Kennedy syndrome.

6.38 D* A young man who has signs and symptoms of bullous emphysema and hepatomegaly should raise the suspicion of him having α_1-antitrypsin deficiency. α_1-Antitrypsin is a glycoprotein, produced by the liver, that prevents the lung being attacked by proteolytic enzymes. Patients have three main phenotypes, depending on their level of α_1-antitrypsin: PiMM (normal homozygous), PiMZ (heterozygous deficient) and PiZZ (homozygous deficient). Of PiZZ patients, 60% will develop panacinar-type emphysema and 12% will develop liver cirrhosis, for which the only curative treatment is liver transplantation. Fortunately the recipient's phenotype changes to that of the donor liver so that this produces normal α_1-antitrypsin. The patient is likely to have an 'obstructive' lung function pattern. All respiratory infections should be treated promptly, so influenza vaccination is prudent.

6.39 E** A history of a malabsorption syndrome associated with polyarthritis, lymphadenopathy, pleural effusions and hyperpigmented skin suggests Whipple's disease. It is a systemic disorder caused by the Gram-positive bacterium *Tropheryma whippelii*. The disease may also affect the heart, central nervous system, causing dementia and nerve lesions, and kidney, resulting in interstitial nephritis. Amyloidosis would be unusual without a history of myeloma or rheumatoid arthritis. Carcinoid is associated with flushing and diarrhoea and not arthritis. There is nothing to suggest inflammatory bowel disease, so ankylosing spondylitis would be unlikely.

6.40 E* Schatzki ring is a benign mucosal ring that occurs at the squamocolumnar junction. Its exact aetiology is unknown but patients typically present with intermittent dysphagia for solid foods, made worse by anxiety or hurrying a meal. As it is a fixed lesion this would differentiate it from problems with peristalsis and oesophageal motility.

6.41 C, H* The scan shows a right chronic subdural haematoma in the frontal lobe. In the right temporal lobe is a high density lesion consistent with an acute intracerebral haemorrhage. There is no midline shift.

6.42 A*** This photograph shows characteristic red-blue plaques over the knuckles and metacarpophalangeal joints, as well as ragged cuticles and dilated nailfold capillaries. Dermatomyositis is also associated with a heliotrope, erythematous rash that also involves the eyelids. Systemic lupus erythematosus is associated with a 'butterfly' rash on the face but this typically spares the eyelids, and on the hands often spares the knuckles.

6.43 D** A young woman presents with headaches, severe hypertension, palpitations and sweating. This could be caused by thyrotoxicosis but the thyroid function tests are normal and she is clinically euthyroid. Hypertension that is resistant to antihypertensives should always raise the possibility of a phaeochromocytoma. Ninety per cent of phaeochromocytomas arise as tumours of the adrenal medulla and secrete amines and peptides, including catecholamines like adrenaline (epinephrine), noradrenaline (norepinephrine) and dopamine. The diagnostic tests of choice would be 24-hour urinary catecholamines and imaging with CT, MRI or MIBG scan to localise the tumour.

6.44 C** The history is suggestive of severe colitis. In the acute setting he will require intravenous hydrocortisone, not oral steroids. In time, full colonoscopy will be necessary to establish the extent of the disease, but there is a higher risk of perforation if it is attempted while the patient is in this state. It would be much safer to do a flexible sigmoidoscopy and gather diagnostic biopsies but treatment should not be delayed. There is a significant risk that this patient will require surgery and so early referral is necessary. A CRP >45 on day 5 postadmission is associated with an increased risk of the patient requiring a colectomy.

6.45 D** This patient complains of abnormal daytime somnolence, cataplexy (episodes of muscular weakness) and paralysis (inability to move during sleep). All these are consistent with narcolepsy. Also associated with narcolepsy are hypnagogic hallucinations, which are hallucinations that typically occur during the sleep–wake transition. Bruxism is forcible teeth grinding that usually occurs at night.

6.46 B*** The X-ray shows a skull with multiple lytic lesions consistent with multiple myeloma. Compare and contrast this image with that of (**2.44**) and (**6.50**).

6.47 A*** This patient has Ehlers–Danlos syndrome. The skin has unusual elasticity in that it can be lifted up from its supporting tissues and springs back again on release. Cutis laxa is where the skin lacks elasticity and hangs in loose folds. Dermatographia is where touching or slightly scratching the skin causes raised reddish marks. Nikolsky's sign (**1.47**) and pathergy (**3.42**) are discussed elsewhere.

6.48 C* This patient develops symptoms and signs of hyperthyroidism postpartum. She has a painless smooth goitre and she is biochemically hyperthyroid. She has no recent illnesses and her ESR is normal, thereby making de Quervain's thyroiditis unlikely. In Graves' disease and toxic solitary adenoma there is increased uptake in the radioactive iodine scan. Postpartum thyroiditis can be a form of autoimmune thyroiditis. During pregnancy there is partial suppression of the immune system. After delivery there can be a dramatic increase in thyroid hormones. The clinical picture may follow a hyperthyroid phase, then a hypothyroid phase, followed by a euthyroid state.

6.49 C* A patient who is requiring repeated drainage of ascites due to a liver disorder should be considered for liver transplantation. Contraindications to liver transplantation include: extrahepatic malignancy; extrahepatic sepsis;

severe portal vein and superior mesenteric vein thrombosis; severe pulmonary hypertension; and development of the acquired immune deficiency syndrome (AIDS).

6.50 D* The patient has a history of headaches and epilepsy. The skull X-ray reveals intracranial 'tramline' calcification of the occipital lobe consistent with Sturge–Weber syndrome.

6.51 D* This patient has Addison's disease, as evidenced by his collapse, low blood pressure, hypoglycaemia, hyponatraemia and hyperkalaemia. He also has buccal mucosa pigmentation. The low calcium and PTH along with the symptoms of tetany are due to hypoparathyroidism. APS type I is a disorder that usually manifests itself in childhood. It requires the combination of two of the following: hypoparathyroidism, adrenal insufficiency and chronic mucocutaneous candidiasis. Other endocrine diseases can also be associated with this syndrome, such as gonadal failure, thyroid disease and type I diabetes.

6.52 E** The history is suggestive of irritable bowel syndrome. The Rome II criteria for the diagnosis of irritable bowel syndrome consider all of the above answers. Most patients with this syndrome do not wake up from sleep to open their bowels; their symptoms are typically worse in the morning when they may open their bowels a number of times. Other symptoms that would be unusual include the passage of blood, weight loss, anaemia and change in bowel habit.

Rome II: A Multinational Consensus Document on Functional Gastrointestinal Disorders. *Gut.* Sep 1999: 45 Supplement II.

6.53 C** Patients with IgA nephropathy tend to present with synpharyngetic haematuria, in that the renal problem occurs at about the same time as the streptococcal infection. There is no evidence of systemic vasculitis and so this cannot be HSP; IgA nephropathy is a limited version of HSP. Acute interstitial nephritis tends to present with fever, arthralgia, skin rash, decreased renal function and eosinophilia; urinalysis would show blood and protein. Epstein–Barr virus infection does not cause haematuria.

6.54 A*** The blood film shows the characteristic intracellular ring trophozites. Of all the options, this is the only one that shows intracellular organisms.

6.55 C** This biopsy is of the liver and shows cirrhosis. There are nodules, which stain deep pink, and surrounding fibrosis, which stains blue. The Childs–Pugh scoring system is used to determine prognosis with cirrhosis.

Score	1	2	3
Albumin	>35	28–35	<28
Ascites	None	Mild	Moderate
Bilirubin	<35	35–50	>50
Encephalopathy	None	Grade I–II	Grade III–IV
Prothrombin time (above control/s)	1–4	4–6	>6

Childs A = 5–6; B = 7–9; C = 10–15: Operative mortality: A = 10%; B = 30%; C = 75%.

Ann Arbor is associated with Hodgkin's lymphoma staging; Rockall's criteria is associated with severity of upper gastrointestinal bleeding; Dukes is concerned with colorectal carcinoma staging; and Breslow's thickness is associated with depth of invasion of malignant melanoma.

6.56 D* This patient has a neutropenic sepsis, probably following his chemo-therapy. The normal neutrophil count is $1.5–7 \times 10^9$/L. He is most at risk of sepsis from *Pseudomonas* sp., staphylococci, *Escherichia coli* and *Klebsiella* sp. Management of such patients includes isolation in a side room and avoidance of contact with individuals with infections; scrupulous hand washing should be undertaken and gloves and aprons put on before entering the room. First-line antibiotic treatment should be aimed at treating these organisms and tazocin and an aminoglycoside like gentamicin would be the best options. Persistent pyrexia may be due to fungal infection but fluconazole should not be started first line in a patient with no evidence of candidiasis.

6.57 C** The blood film shows purple 'smear' or 'smudge' lymphocytes characteristic of chronic lymphocytic leukaemia. Acute lymphoblastic leukaemia is associated with large, round lymphocytes with very little cytoplasm. Lymphocytes in acute myeloid leukaemia are larger but are not always round, and have granular cytoplasm, which may contain Auer rods. Chronic myeloid leukaemia is often characterised by seeing a number of different cells in varying degrees of maturation: basophils, myelocytes, metamyelocytes and blasts. Infectious mononucleosis is characterised by 'atypical' lymphocytes that have a cytoplasm which is pushed out towards the rim and has a tendency to 'stream' around adjacent red cells.

6.58 D* This patient probably has renal artery stenosis, as suggested by unilateral small kidney on ultrasound, bilateral femoral bruits, hypercholesterolaemia, hypertension and renal impairment. The gold standard test for diagnosing this is renal angiography but magnetic resonance angiography could also diagnose the condition. Doppler ultrasound would help identify whether the blood vessels were patent. DMSA scans look for renal scarring. MAG 3 scans are used to see if there is divided function between left and right kidney.

6.59 E* All the pathogens may cause diarrhoeal disease in HIV+ patients but at this CD4 count only non-Hodgkin's lymphoma would be a possibility.

All of the others are unlikely to present until the patient has a CD4 count <100.

6.60 D* This patient has familial Mediterranean fever, as characterised by intermittent abdominal and joint pains in a patient of Mediterranean extraction. In general, this is a fairly benign condition but it may lead to amyloidosis and this is the cause of his nephrotic syndrome. Renal biopsy would be the definitive test to establish the cause of his nephrotic syndrome.

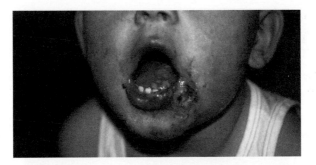

Plate 1.4

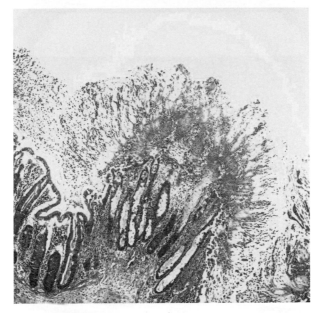

Plate 1.10

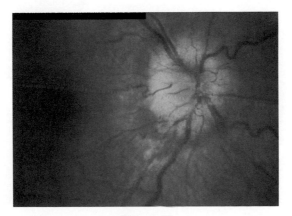

Plate 1.12

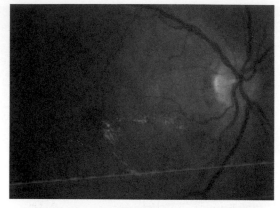

Plate 1.13

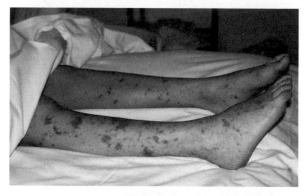

Plate 1.16

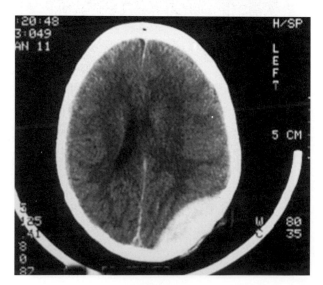

Figure 1.17

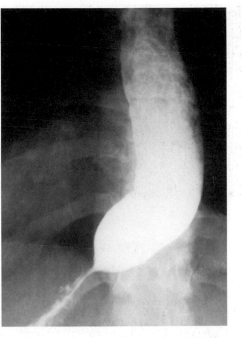

Figure 1.18

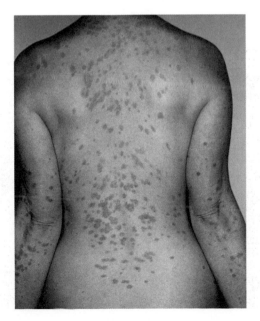

Plate 1.22

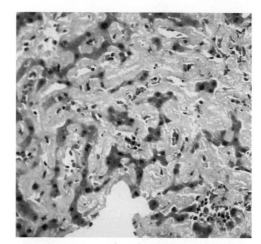

Plate 1.27

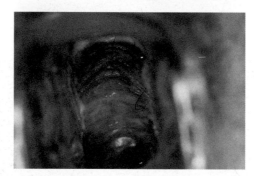

Plate 1.32

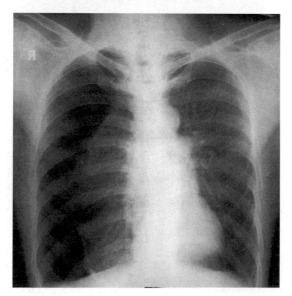

Figure 1.33

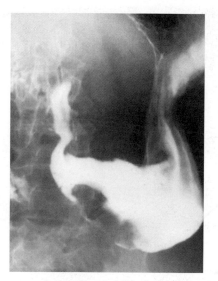

Figure 1.34

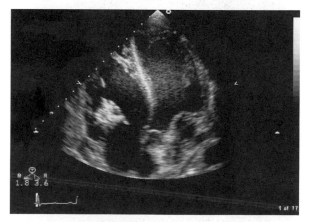

Figure 1.36

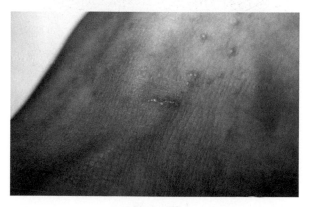

Plate 1.37

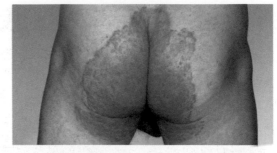

Plate 1.44

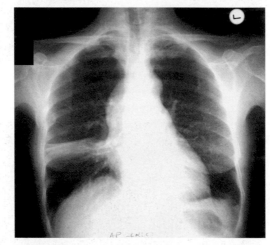

Figure 1.45

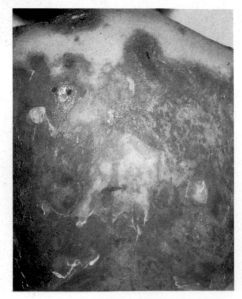

Plate 1.47

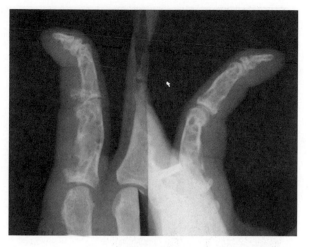

Figure 1.51

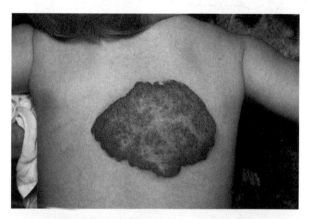

Plate 1.52

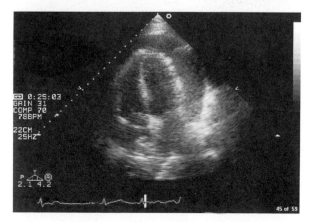

Figure 1.59

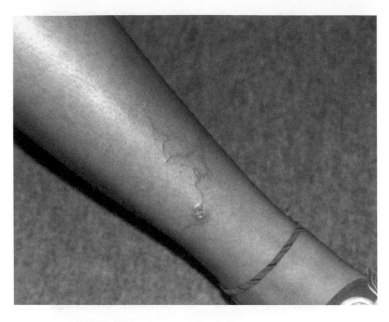

Plate 2.4

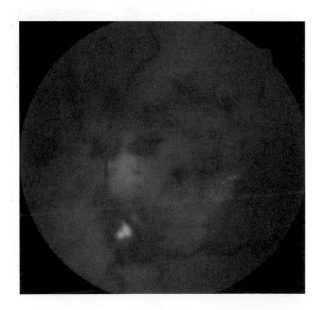

Plate 2.8

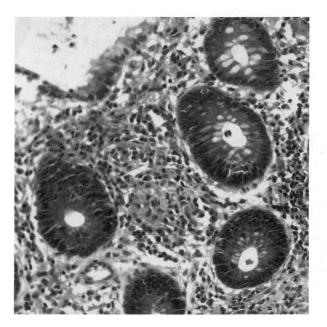

Plate 2.10

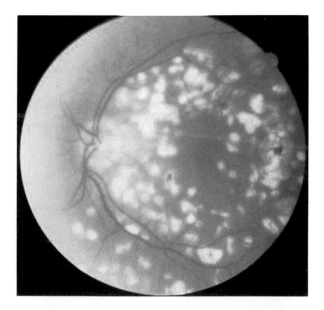

Plate 2.13

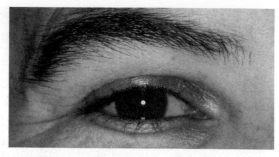

Plate 2.16

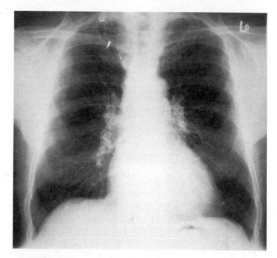

Figure 2.17

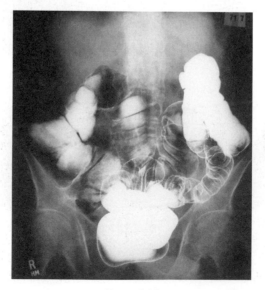

Figure 2.18

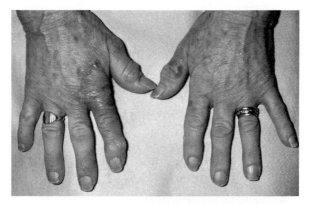

Plate 2.22

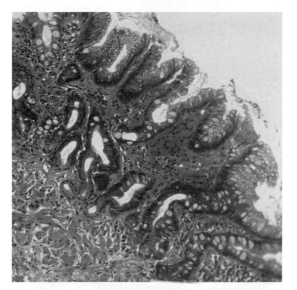

Plate 2.27

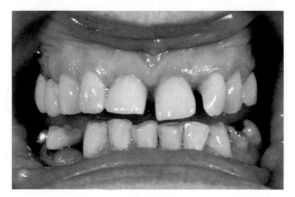

Plate 2.32

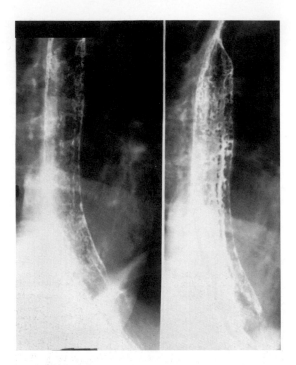

Figure 2.33

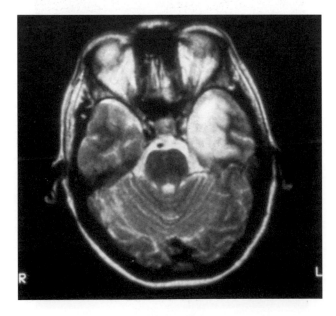

Figure 2.34

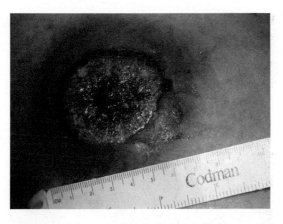

Plate 2.37

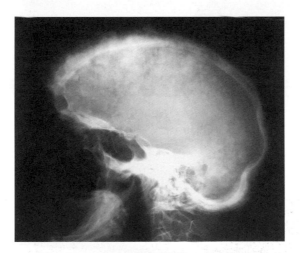

Figure 2.44

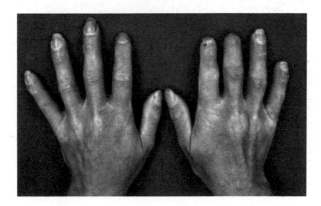

Plate 2.45

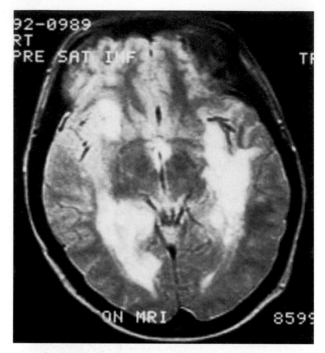

Figure 2.51

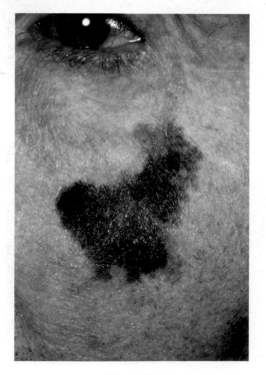

Plate 2.52

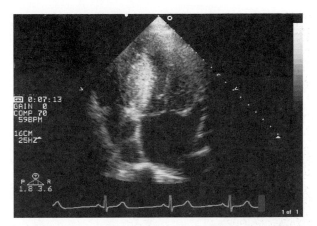

Figure 2.59

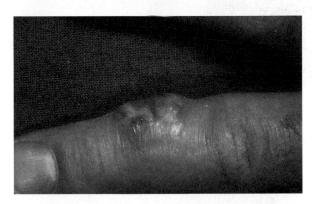

Plate 3.4

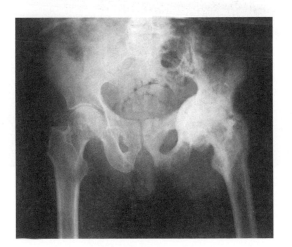

Figure 3.5

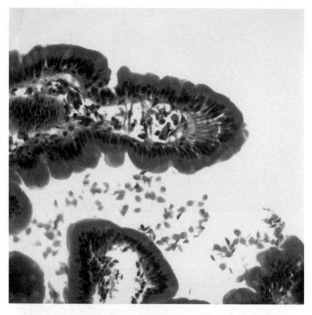

Plate 3.9

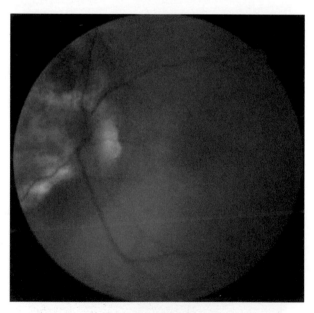

Plate 3.12

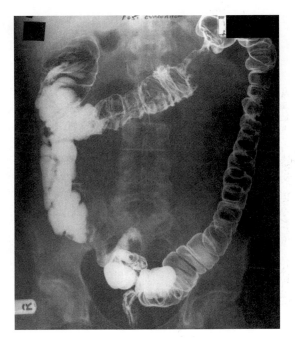

Figure 3.16

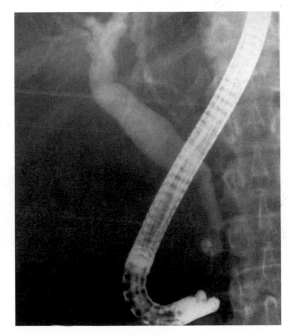

Figure 3.17

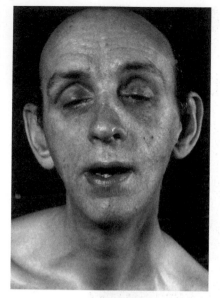

Plate 3.15
(with kind permission from Dr Stuart Coltart)

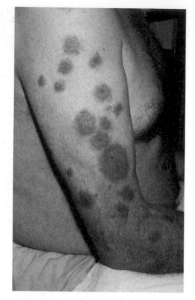

Plate 3.21

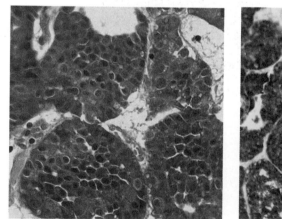

Plate 3.26A

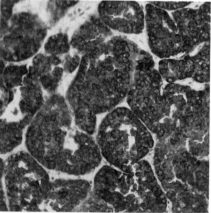

Plate 3.26B

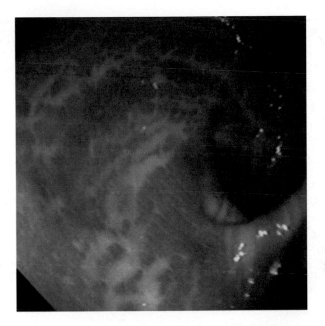

Plate 3.31

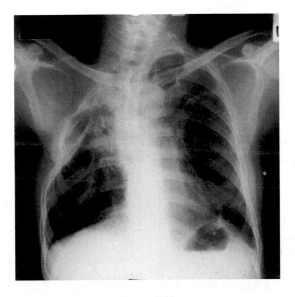

Figure 3.32

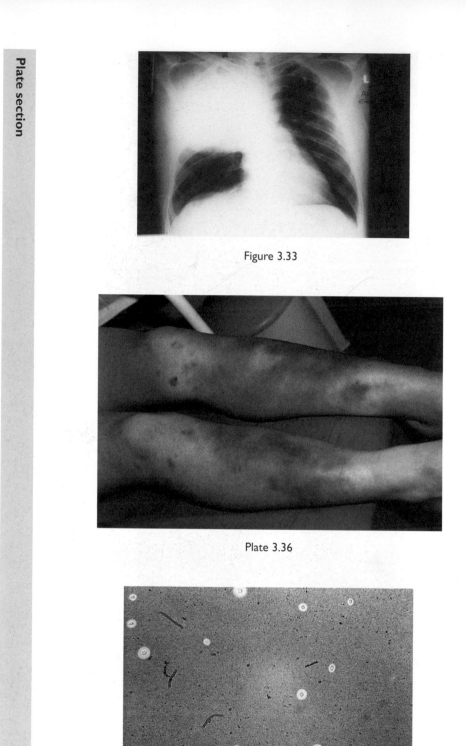

Figure 3.33

Plate 3.36

Plate 3.43

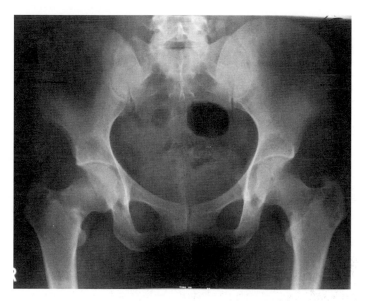

Figure 3.44

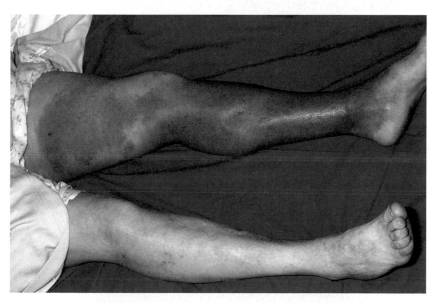

Plate 3.45

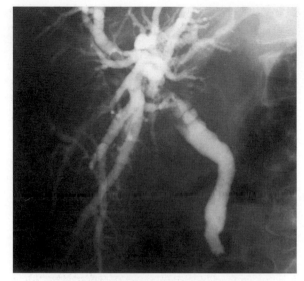

Figure 3.51

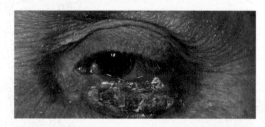

Plate 3.52

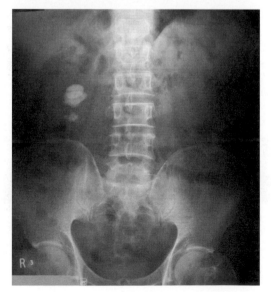

Figure 3.55

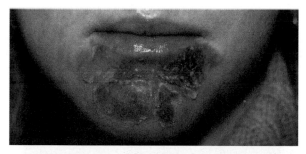

Plate 4.4

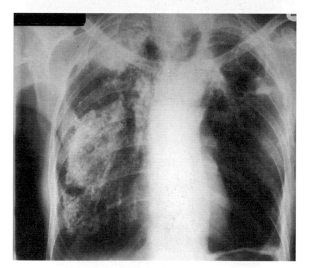

Figure 4.9

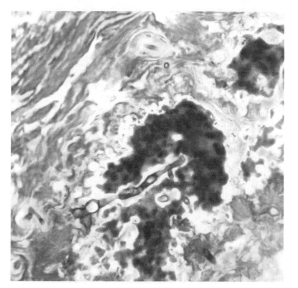

Plate 4.9

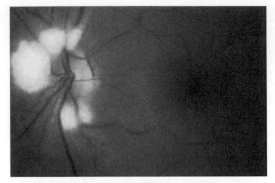

Plate 4.12

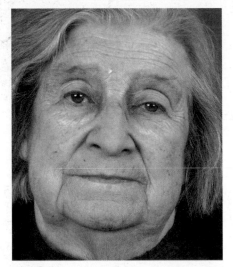

Plate 4.15
(with kind permission from Dr Stuart Coltart)

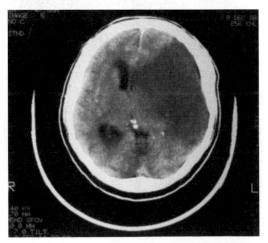

Figure 4.16

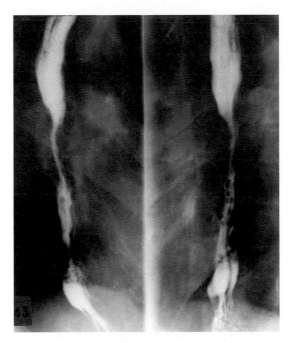

Figure 4.17

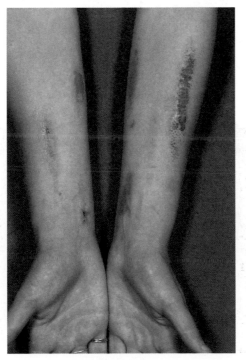

Plate 4.21

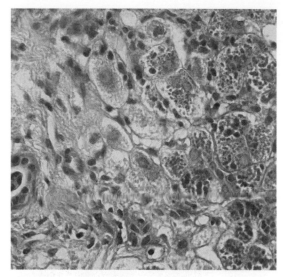

Plate 4.25

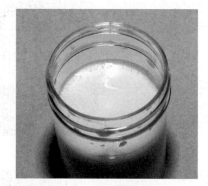

Plate 4.29

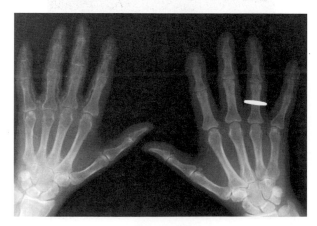

Figure 4.30

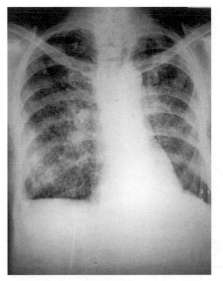

Figure 4.31

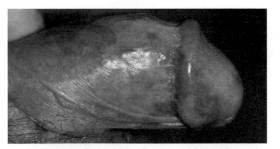

Plate 4.34

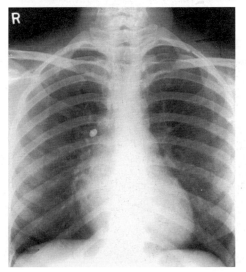

Figure 4.41

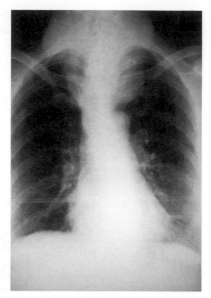

Figure 4.42

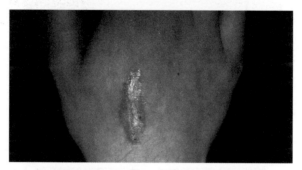

Plate 4.43

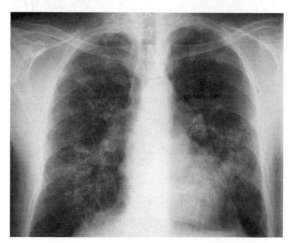

Figure 4.49

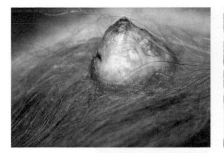

Plate 4.50

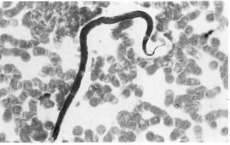

Plate 4.57

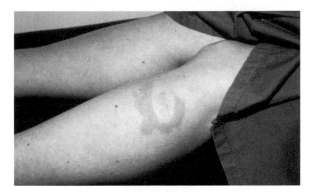

Plate 5.4

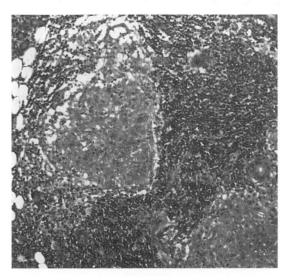

Plate 5.9

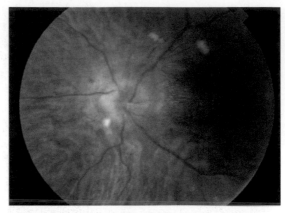

Plate 5.12

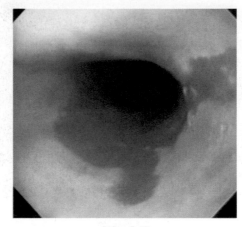

Plate 5.15

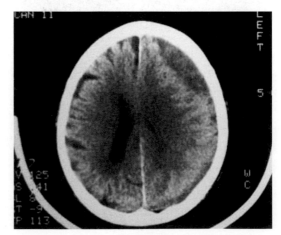

Figure 5.16

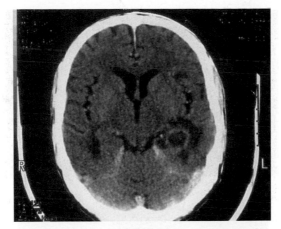

Figure 5.17

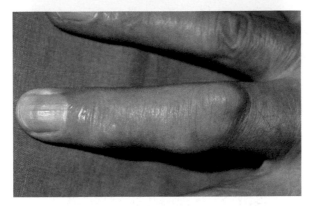

Plate 5.20

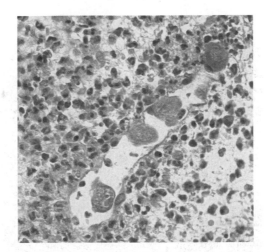

Plate 5.26

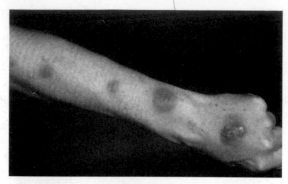

Plate 5.30

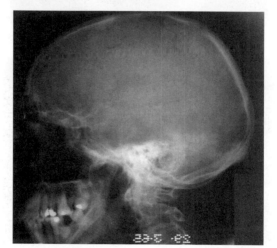

Figure 5.31

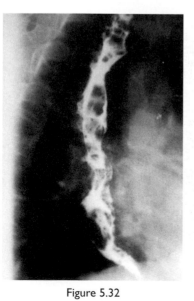

Figure 5.32

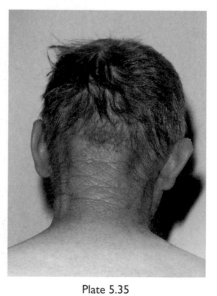

Plate 5.35

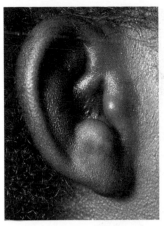

Plate 5.42

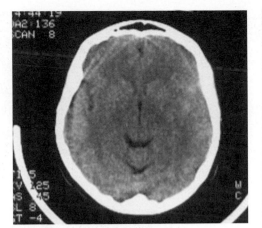

Figure 5.43

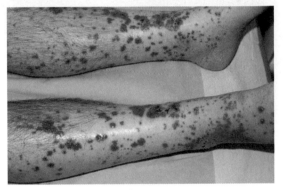

Plate 5.44

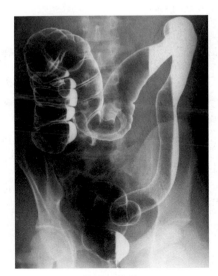

Figure 5.49

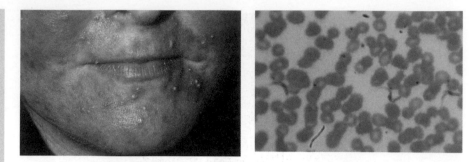

Plate 5.50

Plate 5.57

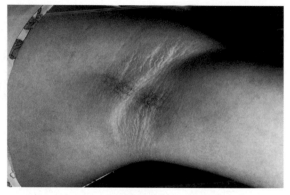

Plate 6.4

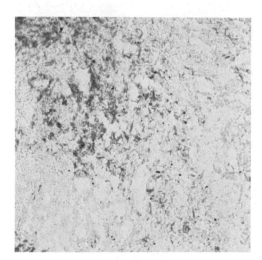

Plate 6.9

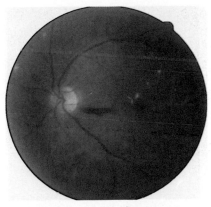

Plate 6.12

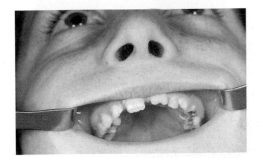

Plate 6.15

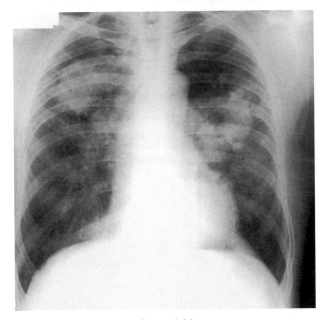

Figure 6.16

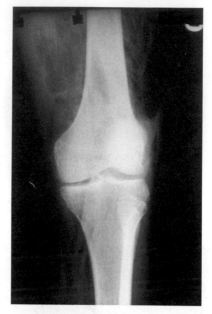

Figure 6.17

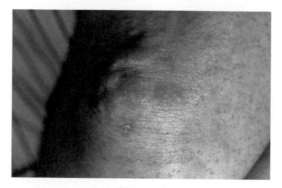

Plate 6.20

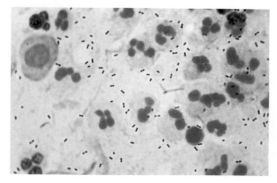

Plate 6.28

294

Malaria Rx

- ABCO$_2$
- Diagnose using multiple thin and thick blood films.
- If unknown or mixed species treat as falciparum.
- Do not use the same medication as used for prophylaxis.

For uncomplicated falciparum:

- Artemether-lumefantrine PO or
- Artesunate-amodiaquine PO or
- Dihydroartemisinin-naphthoquine PO or
- Other artemisinin combination therapy or
- Quinine + doxycycline or clindamycin PO

PTO

- Tepid sponging + paracetamol for fever.

- Transfuse if severe anaemia.

- Consider exchange transfusion if severely unwell.

- Treat algid malaria as per malaria and bacterial shock.

- Monitor TPR, BP, urine output, and blood glucose.

- Daily parasite count, platelets, U+Es and LFTs.

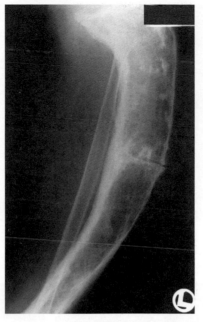

Figure 6.29

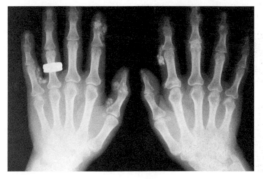

Figure 6.30

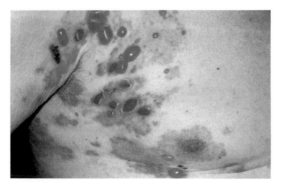

Plate 6.33

Plate 6.40

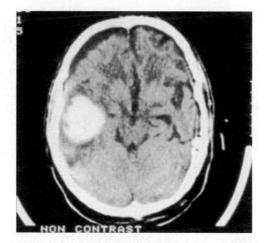

Figure 6.41

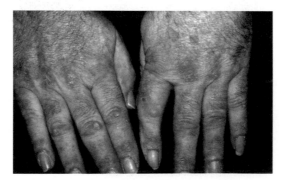

Plate 6.42

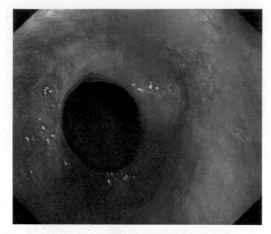

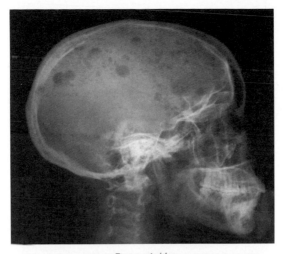

Figure 6.46

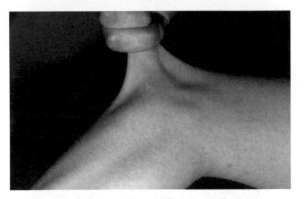

Plate 6.47

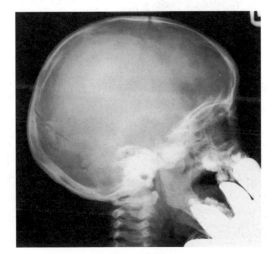

Figure 6.50

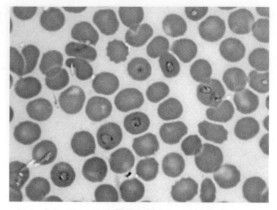

Plate 6.54

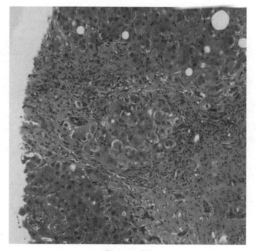

Plate 6.55

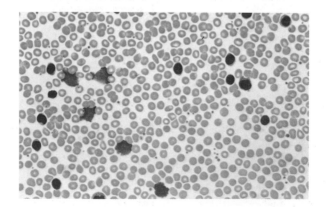

Plate 6.57

Index